BARRON'S

TEAS®

PRACTICE TESTS

LINDA DUNE, Ph.D, RN, CNL

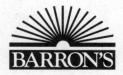

BARRON'S

D1293712

All inquires should be addressed to:
Barron's Educational Series, Inc.
250 Wireless Boulevard
Hauppauge, New York 11788
www.barronseduc.com

ISBN: 978-1-4380-0393-1

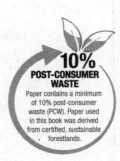

10%
POST-CONSUMER
WASTE
Paper contains a minimum
of 10% post-consumer
waste (PCW). Paper used
in this book was derived
from certified, sustainable
forestlands.

PRINTED IN THE UNITED STATES OF AMERICA
9 8 7 6 5 4

CONTENTS

PRACTICE TEST 4

PRACTICE TEST 5

Introduction

IS THIS BOOK FOR YOU?

How do you know if you should study and practice the tests within this review book? Many nursing programs will make an admission offer based on your grades in the required pre-requisite courses for nursing and the results of the Test of Essential Academic Skills-fifth version (TEAS-V). This test is provided by Assessment Technologies Institute (ATI). Make sure you are studying for the correct test required by the school to which you are applying. There may be other tests required in the nursing program you have chosen. Check your chosen school's website or call their admissions office for admission requirements. The required pre-entrance test is determined by the nursing program and will be listed in those requirements. You know this book is for you if you want to achieve the highest possible score on this extremely important TEAS-V admission evaluation for nursing schools.

Nursing programs have benchmark expectations of minimal scores that predict success, such as certain comprehensive total score and a high score in one or more of the subject specific exam sections. This manual provides you with five practice tests with answer explanations in all subject areas of the TEAS-V. Each of these practice exams have suggested completion times, so that you can review your performance and ability to complete the tests within the time given for the proctored TEAS-V.

ABOUT THE TEST

TEAS-V exam is a test of your knowledge in Reading, Mathematics, Science, and English Language Usage. These four subject areas are identified by nurse educators as most relevant to nursing program success. Each area is subdivided into 12 sub-content areas

- Paragraph Passage Comprehension
- Informational Source Comprehension
- Numbers and Operations
- Data Interpretation
- Algebraic Applications
- Scientific Reasoning
- Human Body Science
- Life Science
- Earth and Physical Science
- Grammar and Word Meaning in Context
- Spelling and Punctuation
- Structure

The exam questions ask for the best answer of four-option, multiple-choice responses. The tests in this book are modeled to emulate the actual testing experience. The actual test is administered with time constraints of 1.3 minutes per question on average. There are a total of 170 questions in each practice exam. The TEAS-V has the same number of questions but 20 of the questions are possible future exam items that are being evaluated and are not counted toward your score. You will not be able to identify these experimental questions, so you must answer all questions with equal concentration.

The TEAS-V is a proctored exam and you must test at an approved testing site. You must schedule and take the exam before the deadline established by your chosen nursing program. To schedule an exam you must log in to the ATI website and set up an account. Make sure you remember your user name and password, because you will need it to sign on to the exam site when you arrive to take the exam. When you register, make sure you identify the nursing program(s) of your preference. If you have applied for multiple programs, you can pay for an additional transcript service ($22 each) so all your schools can view your scores immediately. Many programs will restrict the numbers of attempts at obtaining a successful level on the pre-entrance exam. Check with your chosen program for further information.

USING THIS BOOK

Plan your strategy! Your success will depend upon your effective use of time up to your scheduled exam date. Start early with a study schedule and stick to it. Your goal is to complete all five practice exams in this book with progressively higher scores. The more often you review a weak section, the more likely it will be that your ability to answer the question will increase the next time you see that piece of information. Take each practice exam within the time frame established in the section instructions. Do not go over the stipulated time. Count your actual score and determine your weakest and strongest content areas. Review each question you missed and the answer explanation. If the content is beyond your comprehension, then you may want to review the content area online, in a subject review book, or in a recent textbook on the sub-content area. You want to score higher on each consecutive practice test in this book to become proficient in the required knowledge tested on the TEAS-V exam.

REMEMBER

You will be tested on your knowledge of the topics and your ability to analyze information. Your ability to analyze each subject-focused question demonstrates to the program admission committee that you know the necessary content in order to be successful, you have high-level analysis skills, and you can follow instructions. As a nurse, you are expected to provide reasons or rationales for your actions. Nursing programs are looking for future students who can comprehend and analyze information. Nursing schools want to select students who will be able to complete the program and, therefore, increase the number of qualified nurses in the field. The sub-content areas are there to help the admission committee make a decision about your ability to succeed in the school you have chosen. If you are able to recall facts and definitions along with analyzing and answering test questions correctly, you are well on your way to success!

Practice
TEST 1

ANSWER SHEET
Practice Test 1

READING

1. Ⓐ Ⓑ Ⓒ Ⓓ	13. Ⓐ Ⓑ Ⓒ Ⓓ	25. Ⓐ Ⓑ Ⓒ Ⓓ	37. Ⓐ Ⓑ Ⓒ Ⓓ
2. Ⓐ Ⓑ Ⓒ Ⓓ	14. Ⓐ Ⓑ Ⓒ Ⓓ	26. Ⓐ Ⓑ Ⓒ Ⓓ	38. Ⓐ Ⓑ Ⓒ Ⓓ
3. Ⓐ Ⓑ Ⓒ Ⓓ	15. Ⓐ Ⓑ Ⓒ Ⓓ	27. Ⓐ Ⓑ Ⓒ Ⓓ	39. Ⓐ Ⓑ Ⓒ Ⓓ
4. Ⓐ Ⓑ Ⓒ Ⓓ	16. Ⓐ Ⓑ Ⓒ Ⓓ	28. Ⓐ Ⓑ Ⓒ Ⓓ	40. Ⓐ Ⓑ Ⓒ Ⓓ
5. Ⓐ Ⓑ Ⓒ Ⓓ	17. Ⓐ Ⓑ Ⓒ Ⓓ	29. Ⓐ Ⓑ Ⓒ Ⓓ	41. Ⓐ Ⓑ Ⓒ Ⓓ
6. Ⓐ Ⓑ Ⓒ Ⓓ	18. Ⓐ Ⓑ Ⓒ Ⓓ	30. Ⓐ Ⓑ Ⓒ Ⓓ	42. Ⓐ Ⓑ Ⓒ Ⓓ
7. Ⓐ Ⓑ Ⓒ Ⓓ	19. Ⓐ Ⓑ Ⓒ Ⓓ	31. Ⓐ Ⓑ Ⓒ Ⓓ	43. Ⓐ Ⓑ Ⓒ Ⓓ
8. Ⓐ Ⓑ Ⓒ Ⓓ	20. Ⓐ Ⓑ Ⓒ Ⓓ	32. Ⓐ Ⓑ Ⓒ Ⓓ	44. Ⓐ Ⓑ Ⓒ Ⓓ
9. Ⓐ Ⓑ Ⓒ Ⓓ	21. Ⓐ Ⓑ Ⓒ Ⓓ	33. Ⓐ Ⓑ Ⓒ Ⓓ	45. Ⓐ Ⓑ Ⓒ Ⓓ
10. Ⓐ Ⓑ Ⓒ Ⓓ	22. Ⓐ Ⓑ Ⓒ Ⓓ	34. Ⓐ Ⓑ Ⓒ Ⓓ	46. Ⓐ Ⓑ Ⓒ Ⓓ
11. Ⓐ Ⓑ Ⓒ Ⓓ	23. Ⓐ Ⓑ Ⓒ Ⓓ	35. Ⓐ Ⓑ Ⓒ Ⓓ	47. Ⓐ Ⓑ Ⓒ Ⓓ
12. Ⓐ Ⓑ Ⓒ Ⓓ	24. Ⓐ Ⓑ Ⓒ Ⓓ	36. Ⓐ Ⓑ Ⓒ Ⓓ	48. Ⓐ Ⓑ Ⓒ Ⓓ

MATHEMATICS

1. Ⓐ Ⓑ Ⓒ Ⓓ	10. Ⓐ Ⓑ Ⓒ Ⓓ	19. Ⓐ Ⓑ Ⓒ Ⓓ	28. Ⓐ Ⓑ Ⓒ Ⓓ
2. Ⓐ Ⓑ Ⓒ Ⓓ	11. Ⓐ Ⓑ Ⓒ Ⓓ	20. Ⓐ Ⓑ Ⓒ Ⓓ	29. Ⓐ Ⓑ Ⓒ Ⓓ
3. Ⓐ Ⓑ Ⓒ Ⓓ	12. Ⓐ Ⓑ Ⓒ Ⓓ	21. Ⓐ Ⓑ Ⓒ Ⓓ	30. Ⓐ Ⓑ Ⓒ Ⓓ
4. Ⓐ Ⓑ Ⓒ Ⓓ	13. Ⓐ Ⓑ Ⓒ Ⓓ	22. Ⓐ Ⓑ Ⓒ Ⓓ	31. Ⓐ Ⓑ Ⓒ Ⓓ
5. Ⓐ Ⓑ Ⓒ Ⓓ	14. Ⓐ Ⓑ Ⓒ Ⓓ	23. Ⓐ Ⓑ Ⓒ Ⓓ	32. Ⓐ Ⓑ Ⓒ Ⓓ
6. Ⓐ Ⓑ Ⓒ Ⓓ	15. Ⓐ Ⓑ Ⓒ Ⓓ	24. Ⓐ Ⓑ Ⓒ Ⓓ	33. Ⓐ Ⓑ Ⓒ Ⓓ
7. Ⓐ Ⓑ Ⓒ Ⓓ	16. Ⓐ Ⓑ Ⓒ Ⓓ	25. Ⓐ Ⓑ Ⓒ Ⓓ	34. Ⓐ Ⓑ Ⓒ Ⓓ
8. Ⓐ Ⓑ Ⓒ Ⓓ	17. Ⓐ Ⓑ Ⓒ Ⓓ	26. Ⓐ Ⓑ Ⓒ Ⓓ	
9. Ⓐ Ⓑ Ⓒ Ⓓ	18. Ⓐ Ⓑ Ⓒ Ⓓ	27. Ⓐ Ⓑ Ⓒ Ⓓ	

SCIENCE

1. Ⓐ Ⓑ Ⓒ Ⓓ
2. Ⓐ Ⓑ Ⓒ Ⓓ
3. Ⓐ Ⓑ Ⓒ Ⓓ
4. Ⓐ Ⓑ Ⓒ Ⓓ
5. Ⓐ Ⓑ Ⓒ Ⓓ
6. Ⓐ Ⓑ Ⓒ Ⓓ
7. Ⓐ Ⓑ Ⓒ Ⓓ
8. Ⓐ Ⓑ Ⓒ Ⓓ
9. Ⓐ Ⓑ Ⓒ Ⓓ
10. Ⓐ Ⓑ Ⓒ Ⓓ
11. Ⓐ Ⓑ Ⓒ Ⓓ
12. Ⓐ Ⓑ Ⓒ Ⓓ
13. Ⓐ Ⓑ Ⓒ Ⓓ
14. Ⓐ Ⓑ Ⓒ Ⓓ

15. Ⓐ Ⓑ Ⓒ Ⓓ
16. Ⓐ Ⓑ Ⓒ Ⓓ
17. Ⓐ Ⓑ Ⓒ Ⓓ
18. Ⓐ Ⓑ Ⓒ Ⓓ
19. Ⓐ Ⓑ Ⓒ Ⓓ
20. Ⓐ Ⓑ Ⓒ Ⓓ
21. Ⓐ Ⓑ Ⓒ Ⓓ
22. Ⓐ Ⓑ Ⓒ Ⓓ
23. Ⓐ Ⓑ Ⓒ Ⓓ
24. Ⓐ Ⓑ Ⓒ Ⓓ
25. Ⓐ Ⓑ Ⓒ Ⓓ
26. Ⓐ Ⓑ Ⓒ Ⓓ
27. Ⓐ Ⓑ Ⓒ Ⓓ
28. Ⓐ Ⓑ Ⓒ Ⓓ

29. Ⓐ Ⓑ Ⓒ Ⓓ
30. Ⓐ Ⓑ Ⓒ Ⓓ
31. Ⓐ Ⓑ Ⓒ Ⓓ
32. Ⓐ Ⓑ Ⓒ Ⓓ
33. Ⓐ Ⓑ Ⓒ Ⓓ
34. Ⓐ Ⓑ Ⓒ Ⓓ
35. Ⓐ Ⓑ Ⓒ Ⓓ
36. Ⓐ Ⓑ Ⓒ Ⓓ
37. Ⓐ Ⓑ Ⓒ Ⓓ
38. Ⓐ Ⓑ Ⓒ Ⓓ
39. Ⓐ Ⓑ Ⓒ Ⓓ
40. Ⓐ Ⓑ Ⓒ Ⓓ
41. Ⓐ Ⓑ Ⓒ Ⓓ
42. Ⓐ Ⓑ Ⓒ Ⓓ

43. Ⓐ Ⓑ Ⓒ Ⓓ
44. Ⓐ Ⓑ Ⓒ Ⓓ
45. Ⓐ Ⓑ Ⓒ Ⓓ
46. Ⓐ Ⓑ Ⓒ Ⓓ
47. Ⓐ Ⓑ Ⓒ Ⓓ
48. Ⓐ Ⓑ Ⓒ Ⓓ
49. Ⓐ Ⓑ Ⓒ Ⓓ
50. Ⓐ Ⓑ Ⓒ Ⓓ
51. Ⓐ Ⓑ Ⓒ Ⓓ
52. Ⓐ Ⓑ Ⓒ Ⓓ
53. Ⓐ Ⓑ Ⓒ Ⓓ
54. Ⓐ Ⓑ Ⓒ Ⓓ

ENGLISH AND LANGUAGE USAGE

1. Ⓐ Ⓑ Ⓒ Ⓓ
2. Ⓐ Ⓑ Ⓒ Ⓓ
3. Ⓐ Ⓑ Ⓒ Ⓓ
4. Ⓐ Ⓑ Ⓒ Ⓓ
5. Ⓐ Ⓑ Ⓒ Ⓓ
6. Ⓐ Ⓑ Ⓒ Ⓓ
7. Ⓐ Ⓑ Ⓒ Ⓓ
8. Ⓐ Ⓑ Ⓒ Ⓓ
9. Ⓐ Ⓑ Ⓒ Ⓓ

10. Ⓐ Ⓑ Ⓒ Ⓓ
11. Ⓐ Ⓑ Ⓒ Ⓓ
12. Ⓐ Ⓑ Ⓒ Ⓓ
13. Ⓐ Ⓑ Ⓒ Ⓓ
14. Ⓐ Ⓑ Ⓒ Ⓓ
15. Ⓐ Ⓑ Ⓒ Ⓓ
16. Ⓐ Ⓑ Ⓒ Ⓓ
17. Ⓐ Ⓑ Ⓒ Ⓓ
18. Ⓐ Ⓑ Ⓒ Ⓓ

19. Ⓐ Ⓑ Ⓒ Ⓓ
20. Ⓐ Ⓑ Ⓒ Ⓓ
21. Ⓐ Ⓑ Ⓒ Ⓓ
22. Ⓐ Ⓑ Ⓒ Ⓓ
23. Ⓐ Ⓑ Ⓒ Ⓓ
24. Ⓐ Ⓑ Ⓒ Ⓓ
25. Ⓐ Ⓑ Ⓒ Ⓓ
26. Ⓐ Ⓑ Ⓒ Ⓓ
27. Ⓐ Ⓑ Ⓒ Ⓓ

28. Ⓐ Ⓑ Ⓒ Ⓓ
29. Ⓐ Ⓑ Ⓒ Ⓓ
30. Ⓐ Ⓑ Ⓒ Ⓓ
31. Ⓐ Ⓑ Ⓒ Ⓓ
32. Ⓐ Ⓑ Ⓒ Ⓓ
33. Ⓐ Ⓑ Ⓒ Ⓓ
34. Ⓐ Ⓑ Ⓒ Ⓓ

Part 1: Reading

Time: 58 minutes
48 questions

QUESTIONS 1 THROUGH 6 ARE BASED ON THE FOLLOWING PASSAGE.

Unconditional

Susan and Tom had known each other for twenty years. They realized a mutual attraction ten years ago. Tom decided five years ago to travel to Africa to dedicate his life to his people and to concentrate in bringing the newest generation into an understanding of cosmic consciousness. When he left, the two of them decided to stay single in case their feelings could be rekindled when Tom returned.

Susan fell in love with another and married before Tom's return. When he returned to his much awaited love interest, he discovered the truth. He was upset with the news and told Susan that he never wanted to see her again since she did not possess any sense of loyalty. Susan responded, "I love you and always will. I feel our relationship is based on an unconditional affection for each other." She kissed him, walked away, and never contacted him again.

1. What does the title of this passage reflect?

    (A) Theme
    (B) Main idea
    (C) Detail
    (D) Topic

2. The author demonstrated what type of writing in this passage?

    (A) Expository
    (B) Narrative
    (C) Persuasive
    (D) Technical

3. What is the logical conclusion of the above passage?

    (A) Words may have varying definitions.
    (B) Emotions are not a part of this passage.
    (C) There are evident gender differences.
    (D) Distance makes the heart grow fonder.

4. What is the purpose of the passage?

   (A) to entertain the reader
   (B) to express feelings
   (C) to inform the reader
   (D) to persuade the reader

5. What is the text structure used in the above passage?

   (A) sequence
   (B) cause and effect
   (C) comparison and contrast
   (D) description

6. Which of these statements is an example of Tom using an opinion?

   (A) He discovered the truth.
   (B) He was upset with the news.
   (C) He never wanted to see her again.
   (D) He felt she did not have a sense of loyalty.

QUESTIONS 7 THROUGH 11 ARE BASED ON THE FOLLOWING PASSAGE.

Traditional Chinese Medicine

According to Traditional Chinese Medicine (developed over 4000 years ago), a balance of *yin* and *yang* is extremely important to maintain one's health. Yin represents all things that are passive and cold, while yang represents activity and heat. Both of these should be in balance if the *qi* or "energy" of the body is to be maintained to ward off illnesses. According to the Chinese, medication also can have a cold or hot effect on the body. So, when a doctor prescribes a certain medicine, a Chinese patient may not take the complete medication to "balance out" the yin and yang in the body. He or she may do this without informing the physician, and it could result in deteriorating the health condition. If aware of Chinese culture, the doctor would be in a better position to explain to the patient the importance of taking the full medicine, as prescribed.

7. What is the intent of this passage?

   (A) to entertain the reader
   (B) to express feelings
   (C) to inform the reader
   (D) to persuade the reader

8. What was the author's purpose in writing this passage?

   (A) to explain a topic
   (B) to tell a story
   (C) to convince the reader
   (D) to present precise information

9. Identify rationale for identifying this passage as a secondary source of information.

   (A) This must be the only information source for this tradition.
   (B) It was written hundreds of years after the theory.
   (C) Web site information is always accurate.
   (D) The passage was based on a primary source.

10. What is the text structure of this passage?

   (A) sequence
   (B) cause and effect
   (C) comparison and contrast
   (D) description

11. "According to the Chinese, medication also can have a cold or hot effect on the body." Which choice best describes the content expressed in this quote?

   (A) topic
   (B) supporting detail
   (C) main idea
   (D) theme

Last weekend, I went to the National Association meeting. It took a good deal of planning, fundraising, and organizing to get me there, but I made it. I was really excited to see New Orleans and to meet other students from around the country. And let's be honest, I wanted to try some famous New Orleans gumbo. It was a hectic three days full of career planning, networking with future employers, and listening to presentations. I did enjoy the trip but found that the experience of the travel and the overall workshop was not worth the fundraising and the work it took to get there.

12. What is the author's overall conclusion about this national meeting?

   (A) Networking is a hectic experience.
   (B) There are few advantages to organizational membership.
   (C) The time and work required to attend were not balanced by the benefits.
   (D) The student enjoyed this experience very much.

When the food market revealed on its website last month that it would sell bottles of Whataburger ketchup and mustard in its stores, "it got the most hits of any new product we've ever announced," the chain's director of public affairs said.

13. What is the author's intent in the above passage?

   (A) to inform
   (B) to persuade
   (C) to entertain
   (D) to express feelings

According to ComScore's 2012 U.S. Online Auto Insurance Shopping Report, "nearly seventy percent of shoppers reported getting an online quote." The report also found that "the online channel remains the preferred channel for customers shopping for auto insurance policies." You will have the opportunity to click on the best carrier quotes available in your area.

14. In the above passage, what is the purpose of the statement, "the online channel remains the preferred channel for customers shopping for auto insurance policies"?

    (A) to inform
    (B) to persuade
    (C) to entertain
    (D) to express feelings

Particularly in the second quarter of this year, investors must remain sensitive to economic conditions. Mr. Market's mood fluctuates wildly as improving economic conditions threaten to taper quantitative easing that is the unconventional monetary policy. The scale and duration of bond purchases, the primary component of the Federal Reserve's stimulus program, has defined the post-crisis recovery.

15. What is the overall message to the reader in the above passage?

    (A) The market is stable and the reader should invest now.
    (B) Bonds are a more stable investment than stocks.
    (C) The market fluctuations will continue.
    (D) The Federal Reserve has had little impact on the market.

Two years ago, the governor was at the height of power, driving the state legislature to produce tough new restrictions on abortion, pass new curbs on lawsuits, and enact deep budget cuts. In this session, there was a fall into a more traditional role of encouraging and threatening when necessary, but otherwise compromising with other top leaders. The governor played a major role in halting a bill that would have used increased fees to pay for expanded transportation financing, persuading members to oppose it on the grounds that the legislature should not be asking the citizens to pay more to the state at a time of budgetary surplus.

16. What is the author's purpose for writing the above article?

    (A) to praise the governor's accomplishments
    (B) to persuade the public to donate to the state government
    (C) to give the reader an idea of the legislative process
    (D) to compare legislative sessions in times of decrease and surplus

The candidate, a former six-term U.S. congressman from Virginia, is positioning himself as the truest conservative in the next presidential race. He highlights three issues on his campaign website: defining marriage as a union of one man and one woman; establishing a moratorium on green card admissions to the USA; and limiting campaign donations to $200. The members of his party urge you to vote for this candidate since he is an honest spokesman for the conservative platform.

17. What is the author's purpose in the above text?

    (A) to entertain
    (B) to inform
    (C) to persuade
    (D) to express feelings

Flowers for Jack's Wife

Jack was to mow the grass today but really preferred to admire the wild flowers from the heightening weeds. He frequently has some difficulty with the aging lawn tractor. Last week it would not start. He happily paid the mechanic to replace the battery and spark plug on the aging tractor. As this week progressed, he found that the mower's steering mechanism had rusted through. He had replaced the gas in the tank only to discover that when the steering wheel broke off the frame the tractor tilted and the engine head gasket caught on fire. The entire tractor caught fire fueled by the full gas tank. While the tractor burned, he happily entered the house with a wild flower bouquet for his wife exclaiming, some days it is best to relax and smell the flowers!

18. What is the purpose of this passage?

    (A) to inform
    (B) to persuade
    (C) express feelings
    (D) to entertain

The Hispanic culture is full of wedding traditions that can add depth to the wedding day. An example is the *lazo*, a long strand of rosary beads, placed in a figure eight shape around the necks of the couple after they have exchanged their vows. The symbolism of the lazo is to show the union and protection of marriage. Often, specific members of the wedding party are responsible for "lassoing" the bride and groom together after they kneel for the wedding prayer. Sometimes a white satin cord or rope is draped around the shoulders of the bride and groom. Tradition requires the couple to wear the lasso for the remainder of the service. This act is symbolic of their love, which should bind the couple together every day as they equally share the responsibility of marriage for the rest of their lives.

19. Which type of literature is the above passage most likely from?

    (A) a textbook
    (B) a science fiction novel
    (C) a research journal
    (D) a mystery novel

The following e-mail was sent to a director of human resources from a company employee.

> Grace,
>
> When is the newest director position opening for our division? I would like to suggest Mary as an excellent person for the job. She goes way beyond to help us all in our jobs. Everyone here likes her. Please call her to find out if she would interview for our director.
>
> Thank you,
>
> Susan

20. What is the main purpose of this e-mail?

   (A) The author wants Mary to be hired for the open position.
   (B) The author wants to chat.
   (C) The author disagrees with the current way that people are hired.
   (D) The author wants to be included in decisions involving the division.

21. What is the author's bias regarding the new job?

   (A) There are no biases noted.
   (B) She secretly believes that Mary should be hired.
   (C) She is open about having a bias in favor of Mary as a new director.
   (D) It is difficult to identify the author's bias.

The Cannes Film Festival opened with a more open viewpoint. The dresses worn by judges and women attending the festival have strategic openings as a fashion trend. These openings are a way to show skin in a tasteful and provocative way.

22. What is the meaning of "openings" in the passage above?

   (A) an opening in fabric
   (B) a film viewing
   (C) a new building in Cannes
   (D) how to introduce a new topic in a conversation

23. Read and follow the directions below:
   Begin with the word FALLING.
   Move the letter I to immediately after the F.
   Remove the letter A.
   Remove one L.
   Remove NG.
   Add the letter E to the end of the word.
   What new word has been spelled?

   (A) FAIL
   (B) FALL
   (C) FILE
   (D) FUN

24. A reader is attempting to find information in a book by looking at the Table of Contents. On what page would the information about creating a walkway be located in this book?

    (A) Elegant Symmetry   96

    (B) Organizing Your Project   102

    (C) Laying a Patio   104

    (D) Making Paths and Walkways   108

From: Club, Tina

Sent: Wednesday, May 08, 2013 10:43 AM

Subject: Conference information

Greetings District 29:

This is the May meeting notice and includes information re: The Club conference scheduled for Fall 2013.

District 29 meeting notice: The Club District 29 2012-2013 final meeting scheduled 6 pm Tuesday, May 21 at Giovanni's in Angleton (see attached directions; phone number 333-333-3333).

NEWS from The Club:

The dates and places for the Forces and Factors, Issues and Influencers, formerly the Leadership Conference, have been set. We hope that you all will find a date/place that works for you to attend.

Locations and Dates:

Houston	Nov 6, 2013
Lubbock	Sept 12, 2013
Dallas	Sept 20, 2013
San Antonio	Oct 9, 2013

---

25. According to the above e-mail, when is the event in Angleton?

    (A) May 21

    (B) Sept 12

    (C) Oct 9

    (D) Nov 6

Our Adoption Fees**

PET	AMOUNT
Mixed breed dogs	$110
Purebred dogs	$120
Puppies (age 6 months and under)	$130
Mixed breed cats	$85
Kittens	$90
Purebred cats/kittens	$100
Dogs/Cats 7 years or older	$55

**Adoption of 2 animals = $10 off each adoption fee

26. See the table above. The family is preparing to adopt a pet. The daughter wants a small dog and the mother wants a large pure breed. If they decide on the older dog, how old will the dog need to be to qualify for a discount?

    (A) 6 months
    (B) 2 years
    (C) 7 years
    (D) 10 years

Summer
Low Prices!

Prices good through September 10

Family Favorites

BBQ Sauce
Select varieties 17.5–18 oz.
10 for $10 With Card

Salad Dressing
Select varieties, 16 oz. or Marinades, 12 oz.
2 for $3 With Card

Cheese Bars and Spreads
Select varieties, 6 – 8 oz.
2 for $4 With Card

Juices
Select varieties, 59 oz.
10 for $10 With Card

Produce

Brussels Sprouts
24 oz. $3.99

Fresh Selections Vegetable Tray
40 oz. $7.99

Organic Spring Mix
1 lb. or 20 oz.
Fresh Selections Vegetable Tray
$3.99 With Card

Meat & Seafood

Boneless Chicken Breasts
Sold in 3 lb. Bag
$6.99 With Card

Bratwurst or Italian Sausage
Select Varieties, 18 oz.
$2.99 With Card

Tilapia Fillets Frozen
sold in 2.6 lb. bag
$8.99 With Card

27. Based on the above, which meat or seafood is the most economical?

  (A) pork & beans
  (B) tilapia
  (C) chicken
  (D) bratwurst

➤ **Toys—Retail**

AMERICAN FLYER TRAINS
    CENTRAL TELVSN & TRAINS
      4218 Calumt--------------------WE 2-2946
    DILDINE'S
    Factory Authorized Repair Service
    New & Used-Bought & Sold
      5711 Calumt--------------------WE 2-2495

BABYLAND HIRSCHBERG'S INC
    804 Bway Gary------------------------Turnr 6-3685
CENTRAL TELVSN & TRAINS
    4218 Calumt Av--------------------WE 2-4964
DILDINE'S 5711 Calumt Av---------WE 2-2495
Gentry's Quality Hse
    All Toys-Sptg Gds-Applnces-Discounted
    5 Ridge Rd Munstr-----------------TE 6-5066
Goodyear Service Stores
    5706 Hohman Ave-----------------WE 1-6625

McCAULEY'S VARIETY STORE

COMPLETE LINE OF TOYS — SUNDRIES —
SEWING SUPPLIES — AMERICAN GREETING
CARDS
Open Daily 9 AM to 9 PM
730 173rd---------------------------WE 2-1649

JACK & JILL SHOP
    Complete Year Round Selection
    6342 Ridge Rd Lansng----------GR 4-1100
JOE'S ELECTL SERVICE
    606 Burnhm Av CalCty---------TO 2-4470
Lansing Hdw Co
    3263 Ridge Rd Lansng---------GR 4-2471
LIONEL TRAINS—
    CENTRAL TELVSN & TRAINS
      4218 Calumt Av--------------WE 2-4946
    DILDINE'S
    Factory Authorized Repair Service
    New & Used-Bought & Sold
      5711 Calumt------------------WE 2-2495
PEEWEE'S TOYS & HOBBIES

FREE TOY COUNSELING SERVICE

A Complete year-round Selection of Toys
Crafts & Hobby Supplies — Chemistry Sets
& Replacements — Pools — Wheel Goods

Trains – Hrs. 9:30 to 5:30
Mon. & Fri. 9:30 to 9:00

*Conveniently Located in the Heart of
the Highland Business District*

2835 Highway Ave Highland----TE 8-0663

28. Based on the Yellow Page ad above, what are the last four digits of the phone number for the Lionel Toy Train retailer?

    (A) 1378
    (B) 4946
    (C) 5566
    (D) 6917

```
    A           STORE SERVICES

    ATM          Drug         Seafood

    Bakery       Floral       Sushi

    Bank         Organics     Tickets

    Cosmetics    Pharmacy     Wine
```

B	C	D
Day of The Week	Store Hours	Pharmacy Hours
Sunday	10 AM–8 PM	12 Noon–6 PM
Monday	6 AM –11 PM	9 AM–6 PM
Tuesday	6 AM –11 PM	9 AM–6 PM
Wednesday	6 AM –11 PM	9 AM–6 PM
Thursday	6 AM –11 PM	9 AM–6 PM
Friday	6 AM –11 PM	9 AM–6 PM
Saturday	6 AM –11 PM	9 AM–6 PM

29. Based on the above figure, which section displays the store hours?

(A) A
(B) B
(C) C
(D) D

```
        No-Milk Chocolate Cake

        2 ounces milk chocolate

        2 cups soymilk

        1 cup all purpose wheat flour

        2 medium eggs

        2 tablespoons vegetable oil

        1 teaspoon vanilla
```

30. In the above recipe, which ingredient would not be suitable for someone on a lactose-free diet?

(A) soy milk
(B) eggs
(C) vanilla
(D) milk chocolate

Nutrition Facts

Serving 172 g

Amount Per Serving

Calories 200	Calories from Fat 8
	% Daily Value*
Total Fat 1 g	1%
Saturated Fat 0 g	1%
Trans Fat	
Cholesterol 0 mg	0%
Sodium 7 mg	0%
Total Carbohydrate 36 g	12%
Dietary Fiber 11 g	45%
Sugars 6 g	
Protein 13 g	

Vitamin A	1%	●	Vitamin C	1%
Calcium	4%	●	Iron	24%

*Percent Daily Values are based on a 2,000 calorie diet. Your daily values may be higher or lower depending on your calorie needs.

31. Refer to the above label. A woman is keeping a diary of food and nutrient intake. She decided to consume the entire contents of the food in this package. What should she enter on her diary?

    (A) Calories   300
    (B) Fiber   11 Grams
    (C) Sodium   21 Milligrams
    (D) Sugar   18 Grams

32. A person wants to travel to a new location for vacation. Which information source would give the traveler the most unbiased information about The Isle of Man in Northern Europe?

    (A) an article about the island's political structure
    (B) a travel documentary published in 1970
    (C) a travel handbook for the Islands of Northern Europe published in 2011
    (D) a travel brochure published by the Isle of Man department of tourism

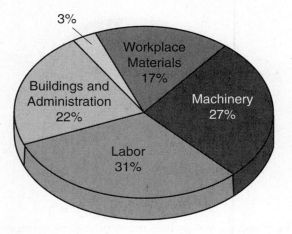

33. The above pie chart was presented to a group of executives wanting to start a new business. They were upset to discover that which one of the categories was highest in expense?

(A) Buildings and Administration
(B) Labor
(C) Other
(D) Machinery

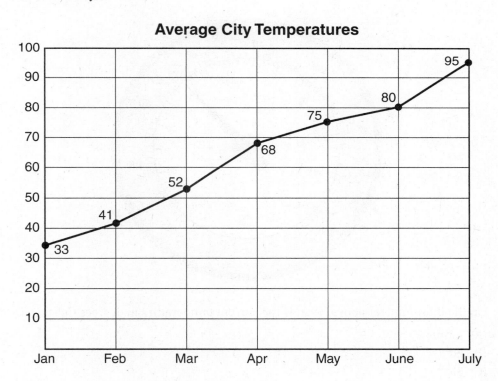

34. Based on the above graph, what is the average increase in temperature per month in this city?

(A) 20°
(B) 15°
(C) 10°
(D) 5°

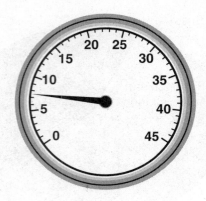

35. A measurement of approximately how many pounds is represented on the scale face above?

   (A) less than 1 pound
   (B) more than 5 pounds
   (C) more than 10 pounds
   (D) exactly 100 pounds

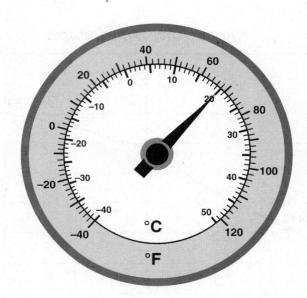

36. On the thermometer above, what is the current temperature in degrees Celsius?

   (A) minus 5°
   (B) 20°
   (C) 35°
   (D) 70°

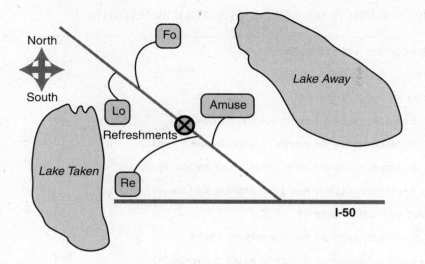

37. Refer to figure above to answer this question. A family has arrived at the park for their day trip. They are entering the park from the south entrance and are traveling north. If they visit each park on their journey, how many times will they pass the refreshment area during their trip?

(A) none
(B) 4
(C) 3
(D) 1

I.   Introductory Statement (hook)

Thesis:

II. Point #1 Topic Sentence

   a. Example (support sentence from book)

   b. Explanation (your words to explain and tie in)

   c. Example (support from research or critical analysis)

   d. Explanation (your words to explain and tie in)

III. Point #2 Topic Sentence

   a. Example (support sentence from book)

   b. Explanation (your words to explain and tie in)

   c. Example (support from research or critical analysis)

   d. Explanation (your words to explain and tie in)

38. Identify a major section of the outline above.

   (A) Sentence Outline Format
   (B) Point #2 Topic Sentence
   (C) Reflecting book strategy
   (D) Example

39. Identify a minor section of the outline above.

   (A) Sentence Outline Format
   (B) Point #2 Topic Sentence
   (C) Reflecting book strategy
   (D) Example

40. The voter has decided to vote in the upcoming elections. Where would the voter find the most unbiased information about the candidate?

   (A) candidatestance.org, all candidate review
   (B) the party's website, the party's candidates
   (C) the opposition's website, the opposing party's website
   (D) the candidate's website, approved by the candidate

Susan responded, "I love you and always will. I feel our relationship is based on an uncondi-tional affection for each other." She kissed him, walked away, and never contacted him again.

41. In the above passage, what is the reason for bolding the name?

    (A) to denote the beginning of a dialogue
    (B) to draw attention to the dialogue
    (C) to identify who is involved in the dialogue
    (D) to denote the ending of the story

42. What is the purpose of the quotation marks in the passage?

    (A) to denote the beginning and end of a statement
    (B) to draw attention to the passage
    (C) to identify an opinion
    (D) to denote the ending of the story

43. What does a thirty percent (30%) chance of rain mean?

    (A) the area will receive thirty percent of the rain
    (B) the area might receive thirty percent of the rain
    (C) the area will expect to be seventy percent dry
    (D) the area has a thirty percent chance of receiving some rainfall

44. The guide words at the top of the page in a phone directory are "Mortgages and Movers." What other business would be found on that page?

    (A) mobile phone
    (B) money transfers
    (C) monuments
    (D) motorcycles

45. The logic seems obvious: Everyone eats food, every day. Food is a massive business. People like having food delivered. And as this company is in both the "massive" and "delivered" businesses, it seems like somewhere we ought to be.

    The phrase, "The logic seems obvious" is reflecting the passage's intent to:

    (A) persuade
    (B) inform
    (C) entertain
    (D) express feelings

46. The following are marathons that have advertised for 2013–2014:

> Fox Valley Marathon + 20 Miler, Half Marathon, Kids Marathon
>
> (St. Charles, IL — 9/22/13)
>
> Fall Foliage Half Marathon + 5K (Lenox, MA — 10/13/13)
>
> Toronto Waterfront Marathon + Half Marathon, 5K
>
> (Toronto, ON — 10/20/13)
>
> Maui Oceanfront Marathon + Marathon Early Start, Half Marathon,
>
> 15K, 10K, 5K (Lahaina, Maui, HI — 1/19/14)
>
> Napa Valley Marathon + 5K (Napa, CA — 3/2/14)

Where is the marathon on October 13, 2013?

(A) Napa Valley

(B) Lenox, MA

(C) Toronto, ON

(D) St. Charles, IL

> Chapter 3 Man: The beginning
>
> 1. When they began
>
> 2. Where they began
>
>   a. Africa
>
>   b. _____
>
>   c. Australia
>
>   d. Europe
>
>   e. North America
>
> 3. How they survived

47. Based on the pattern of the outline above, what is the most reasonable heading for 2. b.?

(A) China

(B) Asia

(C) Mexico

(D) New Zealand

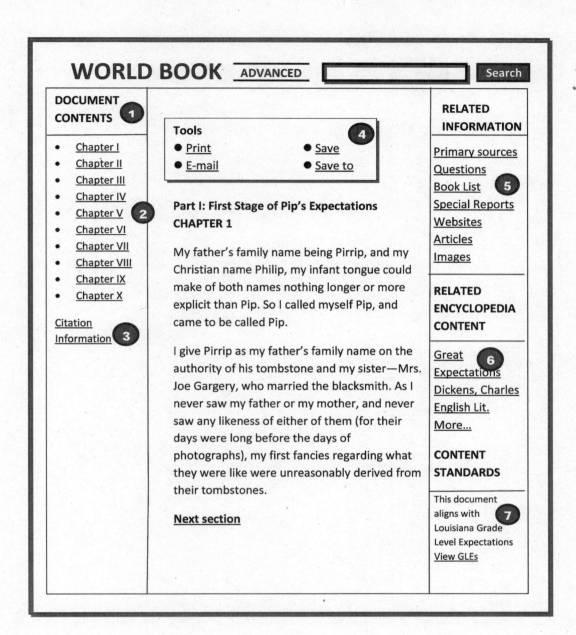

WORLD BOOK ADVANCED | Search

DOCUMENT CONTENTS ❶

- Chapter I
- Chapter II
- Chapter III
- Chapter IV
- Chapter V ❷
- Chapter VI
- Chapter VII
- Chapter VIII
- Chapter IX
- Chapter X

Citation Information ❸

Tools ❹
- Print
- E-mail
- Save
- Save to

Part I: First Stage of Pip's Expectations
CHAPTER 1

My father's family name being Pirrip, and my Christian name Philip, my infant tongue could make of both names nothing longer or more explicit than Pip. So I called myself Pip, and came to be called Pip.

I give Pirrip as my father's family name on the authority of his tombstone and my sister—Mrs. Joe Gargery, who married the blacksmith. As I never saw my father or my mother, and never saw any likeness of either of them (for their days were long before the days of photographs), my first fancies regarding what they were like were unreasonably derived from their tombstones.

Next section

RELATED INFORMATION

Primary sources
Questions
Book List ❺
Special Reports
Websites
Articles
Images

RELATED ENCYCLOPEDIA CONTENT

Great Expectations ❻
Dickens, Charles
English Lit.
More...

CONTENT STANDARDS

This document aligns with ❼ Louisiana Grade Level Expectations
View GLEs

48. Based on the above webpage, identify the section to explore websites related to the novel.

(A) 1 Document Contents
(B) 3 Citation Information
(C) 5 Related Information
(D) 7 Content Standards

Part 2: Mathematics

Time: 51 minutes
34 questions

1. $40 + (4 \times (5+3)^2)$

   Simplify the expression above. What is the correct answer?

   (A) 64
   (B) 88
   (C) 148
   (D) 296

2. What is the solution for $0.114 - 32.22$?

   (A) 31.106
   (B) −32.106
   (C) 32.314
   (D) −33.14

3. Tammy purchased five 29-cent stamps and nine 44-cent stamps. She gave the clerk $10.00. How much change should she receive?

   (A) $1.45
   (B) $3.96
   (C) $4.59
   (D) $6.04

4. What is the sum of $3\frac{1}{2}$ and $6\frac{1}{3}$?

   (A) $6\frac{5}{6}$
   (B) $9\frac{2}{3}$
   (C) $9\frac{5}{6}$
   (D) $10\frac{1}{2}$

5. What is the product of the numbers $0.45 \times \frac{1}{6}$?

   (A) 0.066
   (B) 0.075
   (C) 0.125
   (D) 0.297

6. What is the quotient of 9 divided by $\frac{1}{4}$?

   (A) 0.18
   (B) 1.8
   (C) 3.6
   (D) 36

7. The student enrollment cannot exceed 15 students per 1 faculty proportion. How many faculty members will be needed for a class size of 128 students?

   (A) 6
   (B) 8
   (C) 9
   (D) 12

8. What is the ratio of 30 minutes to 5 hours?

   (A) 1:10 or 1/10
   (B) 1:5 or 1/5
   (C) 1:15 or 1/15
   (D) 1:3 or 1/3

9. Simplify the expression 0.125 divided by 0.2.

   (A) 0.45
   (B) 0.625
   (C) 0.66
   (D) 4.5

10. What is the approximate conversion of the square root of 10 $\left(\sqrt{10} \right)$?

    (A) 2
    (B) 5
    (C) 1
    (D) 3

11. The realtor always collects 8% of the selling price of each home sold by the corporation. The realtor collected $12,100. What was the selling price of the home?

    (A) $142,006
    (B) $151,250
    (C) $240,050
    (D) $360,500

12. Convert $\frac{1}{32}$ into a percent.

   (A) 4%
   (B) 5%
   (C) 2%
   (D) 3%

13. Convert 33% to a fraction.

   (A) $\frac{1}{2}$
   (B) $\frac{1}{7}$
   (C) $\frac{1}{3}$
   (D) $\frac{1}{8}$

14. The enrollment of a college decreased from 1,000 to 890. What is the percentage of decrease?

   (A) 11%
   (B) 15%
   (C) 9%
   (D) 13%

15. Of these numbers, which is the largest?

   (A) $\frac{78}{100}$
   (B) $\frac{2}{3}$
   (C) $\frac{1}{2}$
   (D) $\frac{5}{6}$

16. The trip from New York to Chicago is 792 miles. Estimate the numbers of gallons of gasoline it will take in your rental car that gets 28 miles per gallon.

   (A) 32
   (B) 28
   (C) 20
   (D) 18

17. Reconcile the checking account for this month. The previous balance was $4,250. Deposits were made for $680 and $420. Checks were written for $1,100 and $350. What is the remaining balance?

   (A) $3,900
   (B) $3,000
   (C) $490
   (D) $4,900

18. A couple is planning to purchase a new house. They were told never to let a residence expense exceed 25% of their monthly income. The couple now earns $4125 per month after taxes are deducted from their payroll checks. How much can they afford per month toward this new residence?

    (A) $751
    (B) $985
    ✓ (C) $1031
    (D) $1505

19. An employee received a 2% per week pay increase for performance and overall sales commission. The salary before the increase was $800 per week. What is this employee's annual salary after the 2% increase?

    (A) $50,200
    ✓ (B) $42,432
    (C) $40,618
    (D) $38,164

20. The movie that you rented has the production date in Roman numerals. What is MCMLXXIV in Arabic numerals?

    (A) 1874
    (B) 1924
    (C) 2004
    (D) 1974

21. The runner, new to marathons, is trying to decide if 4 kilometers is beyond the running school training level of 4 miles. What is the distance in miles for this 4-kilometer race?

    (A) 4.25
    ✓ (B) 1.24
    (C) 3.48
    (D) 2.48

22. Convert 2 gallons to liters.

    (A) 2.0
    (B) 7.6
    ✓ (C) 3.8
    (D) 4.5

23. The infant lost one-half pound. What was the decrease in grams?

    (A) 150
    ✓ (B) 224
    (C) 312
    (D) 324

24. How many centimeters are in 2 meters?

    (A) 0.2
    (B) 2.0
    (C) 20
    (D) 200

25. What metric unit of measurement would be best for administering an oral dose of cough medicine?

    (A) deciliter
    (B) kiloliter
    (C) liter
    (D) milliliter

26. On the map key, 1 inch = 150 miles. You measure the distance between Dallas and Chicago as 6.5 inches. Estimate the driving distance in miles.

    (A) 975
    (B) 1,025
    (C) 500
    (D) 650

27. "Physiological aging can be slowed with diet and exercise." If this theory were tested, what would be the independent variable?

    (A) slowed
    (B) physiological
    (C) diet
    (D) aging

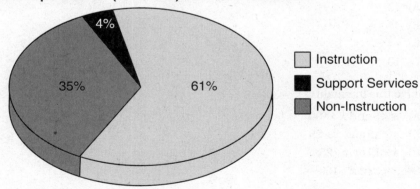

The Cost of an Education: Breakdown of Average Cost Per Student Expenditures (in dollars) for Public Education

4%

35%

61%

Instruction

Support Services

Non-Instruction

NCES Common Core Data (CCD) 2002-03

28. Based on the above pie chart, if school district taxes for your property are $2,000 per year, how much money are you paying for support services and non-instruction per year?

    (A) $500
    (B) $610
    (C) $780
    (D) $1,220

29. The characteristics of a city need to be described. Which chart or graph would best visually represent the information?

   (A) pie chart
   (B) bar chart
   (C) Gantt chart
   (D) histogram

30. Simplify this expression: $(12xy + 8xy^2 - 4xy) \div (24xy)$

   (A) $2y + \dfrac{1}{6}$
   (B) $1xy - 4y$
   (C) $8xy^2 + 1$
   (D) $\dfrac{1}{3}y + \dfrac{1}{3}$

31. Express this case in an algebraic formula. A man is three times his daughter's age plus 5 years. If she is "y" years old, what is his age?

   (A) $3y + 5 = x$
   (B) $5y + 2 = x$
   (C) $2y + 5x = x$
   (D) $2xy - 5 = x$

32. Solve this equation for x: $\dfrac{x}{2} + 5 = 9$

   (A) 4
   (B) 6
   (C) 8
   (D) 16

33. Solve this equation for j: $j + 3 = 7$

   (A) 13
   (B) 4
   (C) -4
   (D) 10

34. Solve this inequality: $[x - 20] > 5$

   (A) $x < 5$ and $x > 100$
   (B) $x < 15$ and $x > 25$
   (C) $x < 15$ or $x > 25$
   (D) $x < 5$ or $x > 100$

Part 3: Science

Time: 66 minutes

54 questions

THE FOLLOWING TWO QUESTIONS ARE BASED ON THE PERIODIC TABLE BELOW.

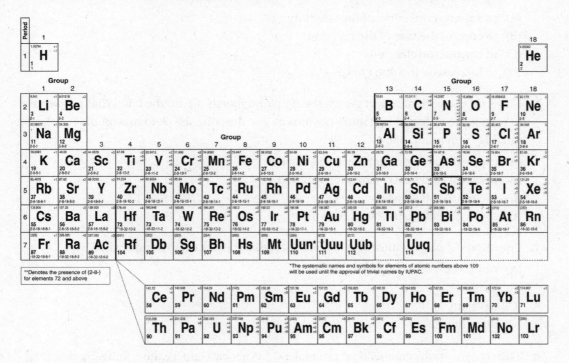

1. How many protons does magnesium (Mg) have?

   (A) 4

   (B) 8

   (C) 12

   (D) 16

2. How many neutrons does an atom of chromium (Cr) contain? The mass number is 52.

   (A) 24

   (B) 12

   (C) 52

   (D) 28

3. When is the potential energy of an amusement ride highest?

   (A) while it is traveling in a circle
   (B) while ascending
   (C) at the bottom of a hill
   (D) at the middle of a hill

4. If an element has an atomic mass of 16 and atomic number of 8, how many electrons are there in the atom if it is neutral?

   (A) 8
   (B) 9
   (C) 24
   (D) 34

5. What is the purpose of a catalyst in a chemical reaction?

   (A) to enhance the effect of the reaction
   (B) to control the rate of the reaction
   (C) to control the electrons
   (D) to increase activation energy

6. Gases on the periodic chart are on the right and metals are on the left. What properties of metals are different and more obvious as you describe the elements on the chart, moving from group 3 to 1?

   (A) they will have stronger electrical current
   (B) they will cool slowly when refrigerated
   (C) they will heat slowly
   (D) they will change in electronegativity

7. The bonds in carbon dioxide (CO_2) are shared. What are these bonds called?

   (A) saturated
   (B) ionic
   (C) covalent
   (D) unsaturated

8. Two oxygen atoms can be joined to make O_2. What can you assume, knowing that this is an ionic bond?

   (A) This is an attraction between similarly charged electrons.
   (B) This is an electron attraction.
   (C) This bond will be difficult to separate.
   (D) This bond is highly volatile.

9. What is the expected product when combining acids and bases?

   (A) energy
   (B) an ionic negative charged salt
   (C) oxygen
   (D) water

10. Suppose you place 200 grams of water to boil. Compute the energy used based on a latent heat of water at 540 calories per gram.

   (A) 540 kilocalories
   (B) 11 kilocalories
   (C) 108 kilocalories
   (D) 210 kilocalories

11. Which is an example of inductive reasoning?

   (A) Patients who have surgery have pain; therefore, all patients who have surgery will need continuous pain medicine.
   (B) This patient has pain and has had surgery; therefore, all patients who have surgery will probably need pain medicine.
   (C) I know several patients who needed pain medicine after surgery, so all patients will need to be medicated.
   (D) Patients, after surgery, will need pain medication.

12. Which of these studies would demonstrate the best research protocol?

   (A) Groups of women with chronic health concerns were randomly divided into a control and intervention group and received an online educational intervention.
   (B) Women with chronic health concerns were recruited for a national study, randomly selected for the study, then randomly divided into a control and intervention group and received an online educational intervention.
   (C) All women with chronic health concerns were randomly divided into a control and intervention group and received an online educational intervention.
   (D) All women with chronic health concerns received an online educational intervention and then were followed over time.

13. How should a researcher test the research question that suggests that eating certain foods decreases headaches?

   (A) Randomly divide study participants into groups, measure the severity of headache pain before providing different foods to each group, and then measure the severity of headaches one hour after the food.
   (B) Have each randomly divided group of study participants consume the same foods every day and follow up after one week.
   (C) Suggest common comfort foods and ask study participants to map their own relief from their headaches.
   (D) Randomly divide study participants into groups, measure the severity of headache pain before providing the same foods to one group, provide a placebo to the other group, and then measure the severity of headaches one hour after the food or placebo was given.

14. Which step would follow problem identification in the scientific process?

   (A) hypothesis testing
   (B) data collection
   (C) analysis of data
   (D) formulating the research question

15. What would give the highest confidence in a theory?

   (A) repeated testing over time
   (B) repeatability
   (C) presence of bias
   (D) reliability of the data

16. Why is scientific research dependent on technology and mathematics?

   (A) Technology helps by placing the information on charts.
   (B) Technology provides descriptions of data.
   (C) Technology and mathematics assist in describing relationships between data sets.
   (D) Technology provides qualitative information.

QUESTIONS 17 THROUGH 19 ARE BASED ON THE FOLLOWING GRAPH.

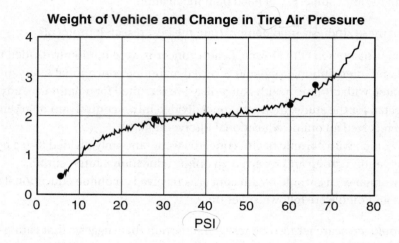

17. According to the above graph, what is suggested about the weight of a vehicle and tire pressure?

   (A) As the vehicle increases in weight there is more pressure on tires.
   (B) As the vehicle decreases in weight there is more pressure on tires. ✗
   (C) There is no relationship between vehicle weight and tire pressure.
   (D) As the vehicle increases in weight there is less pressure on tires.

18. Which one of these statistical terms describes the relationship in the above graph?

   (A) expected
   (B) direct
   (C) indirect
   (D) proportional

19. What is the logical conclusion of the study results in question 17?

    (A) If weight creates an increase in PSI, check the air pressure before driving with a large load.

    (B) There is no relationship, so no need to check the tire pressure.

    (C) Make sure to hyper-inflate all tires for regular driving in case you need to transport heavy loads.

    (D) Under-inflate the tires so you will not have a blowout when transporting heavy loads.

20. The researcher is interested in determining if there is an effect of decreasing test scores and numbers of miles driven per day to class. Decreasing test scores are what type of variable?

    (A) extraneous

    (B) responsive

    (C) dependent

    (D) independent

QUESTIONS 21 AND 22 ARE BASED ON THE FOLLOWING TABLE.

EB VIRUS CULTURE SIZE ON DAY 3, IN CM	ENVIRONMENTAL TEMPERATURE
3	68
5	74
7	82
8	95
9	97
11	98
30	100

21. Several culture tubes, once exposed to the Epstein Barr Virus, were placed in varying environmental temperatures. The data in the above table would suggest what type of relationship between Epstein Barr culture size and environmental temperature?

    (A) proportional

    (B) indirect

    (C) direct

    (D) scattered

22. These same viral cultures were then exposed to disinfectants mixed in water in 1:3, 1:2, and 1:1 water and disinfectant. The kill zone was increased in the 1:3 concentration but not in the others. The experiment was repeated over time with the same virus with the same effect. What should the researcher do next?

(A) Continue repeating the study.
(B) Test progressive concentrations between 1:3 and 1:2 proportions.
(C) Try other disinfectants.
(D) Work with a different virus.

23. An automobile has suddenly stopped on the road and the engine is overheating. What data would convince the driver that it is a broken radiator?

(A) Several hoses are disconnected.
(B) The distributor cap is missing.
(C) The air conditioning is not working.
(D) Steam is escaping from the radiator.

24. What is considered the end of a scientific report on research data?

(A) discussion
(B) analysis of data
(C) research question
(D) problem identification

25. Which human body function provides the essential function of control of body functions through the endocrine system?

(A) adaptation
(B) regulation
(C) elimination
(D) self-duplication

26. The spleen is located in which section of the body?

(A) to the right of the sagittal section
(B) in the dorsal body cavity
(C) in the ventral body cavity
(D) in a superficial section

27. In describing a cut on a finger as compared to a cut present on the forearm, how would the pathologist describe the finger injury?

(A) proximal to the elbow
(B) distal to the wrist
(C) according to a transverse plane
(D) as intermediate to the elbow

28. Where does deoxygenated blood enter the heart?

(A) pulmonary veins
(B) aorta
(C) left atrium
(D) right atrium

29. Which valves are involved in the movement of oxygenated blood?

   (A) tricuspid
   (B) mitral
   (C) portal
   (D) vena cava

30. What happens during the respiratory process of expiration?

   (A) the diaphragm contracts
   (B) oxygen leaves the lungs
   (C) carbon dioxide leaves the lungs
   (D) blood returns to the right side of the heart

31. What is the anatomical structure responsible for internal respiration?

   (A) bronchial tubes
   (B) trachea
   (C) cilia
   (D) alveoli

32. Digestion of proteins occurs primarily in what structure in the digestive system?

   (A) mouth
   (B) stomach
   (C) duodenum
   (D) ileum

33. What anatomical structure in the small intestine increases the ability to absorb nutrients?

   (A) villi
   (B) alveoli
   (C) duodenum
   (D) rugae

34. What is the first bodily defense against invasion of bacteria or viruses?

   (A) antigens
   (B) antibodies
   (C) T-cells
   (D) skin

35. What type of immunity is it when a child develops measles and acquires immunity to future infections?

   (A) active
   (B) passive
   (C) cell-mediated
   (D) artificially acquired

36. Which of the body systems serves as the body's control system?

    (A) lymphatic
    (B) nervous system
    (C) respiratory
    (D) muscular

37. Which human body organ systems are most involved with acid base balance?

    (A) neurologic and skeletal
    (B) digestive and immune
    (C) circulatory and endocrine
    (D) respiratory and urinary

38. What type of country would be most likely to report high fertility rates?

    (A) those in the northern hemisphere
    (B) those in tropical climates
    (C) underdeveloped
    (D) more developed

39. When would you expect overpopulation to occur?

    (A) If the crude birth rate exceeds crude death rate.
    (B) If the crude death rate exceeds birth rate.
    (C) If mortality rates exceed morbidity rates.
    (D) If morbidity rates exceed infant mortality rates.

40. Which human body system utilizes enzymes as a primary role?

    (A) skeletal
    (B) digestive
    (C) endocrine
    (D) respiratory

41. Which organ produces bile, an essential enzyme for the breakdown of fat?

    (A) stomach
    (B) pancreas
    (C) spleen
    (D) gall bladder

42. What major factor influences the population of a country?

    (A) immigration
    (B) resources available
    (C) overpopulation
    (D) morbidity rate

43. What is the purpose of deoxyribonucleic acid (DNA)?

    (A) pentose formation
    (B) phosphate regulation
    (C) adenine base replication
    (D) messenger for reproduction

44. Which of these would be a type of adaptation?

    (A) people who avoid the sea coast after storms
    ✓ (B) birds that fly south to a different place each year
    ✓ (C) resistance to antibiotics developed by some bacteria
    (D) changes in ribonucleic acid (RNA) over a life span

45. Which nucleic acid is not found in RNA but is in DNA?

    (A) thymine
    (B) cytosine
    (C) adenine
    (D) guanine

46. Which eukaryotic cell structure is missing in prokaryotic cells?

    (A) ribosomes
    ✓ (B) nuclear membrane
    (C) flagellum
    (D) cytoplasm

47. What is the unique cellular organelle in plant cells?

    (A) Golgi apparatus
    (B) vacuole
    ✓ (C) chloroplast
    (D) endoplasmic reticulum

48. What is the next step in DNA replication in this sequence?

    G_1, RNA pairing with their DNA partner

    (A) interphase
    (B) G_2
    ✓ (C) mitosis
    (D) S phase

49. Which cells use the process of meiosis as cell replication?

    (A) prokaryotic
    ✓ (B) reproductive
    (C) eukaryotic
    (D) chromosomes

50. Cellular respiration requires which cellular organelle to function?

    ✓ (A) mitochondria
    (B) centrosome
    (C) endoplasm
    (D) ribosome

51. Genetic traits are expressed through which cellular component?

    (A) Golgi apparatus
    (B) proteins
    (C) chloroplasts
    (D) glucose

52. Which cells carry mutations on to future generations?

    (A) gametes
    (B) genome
    (C) germ
    (D) mutant

53. Genetic variations of hair color are a result of which of these genetic codes?

    (A) phenotypes
    (B) genomes
    (C) mutagens
    (D) genotypes

54. What are the possible offspring of the genetic crossing of a homozygous grape (seedless) vine with a heterozygous grape with seeds?

    (A) 25% with seeds
    (B) 75% with seeds
    (C) 25% seedless
    (D) 50% seedless

Part 4: English and Language Usage

Time: 34 minutes

34 questions

1. Jack _____ texted kind words to Jill.

   Which of the following options correctly completes the sentence above?

   (A) scrupulous
   (B) script
   (C) sudden
   (D) suddenly

2. John, upon <u>receiving</u> the startling news, <u>reluctantly</u> cancelled the trip.

   Which of the following correctly identifies the parts of speech in the underlined portions of the sentence above?

   (A) noun; adverb
   (B) noun; adjective
   (C) verb; adverb
   (D) adjective; adverb

3. Which of the following sentences has correct subject–verb agreement?

   (A) When arriving to the restaurant, he find the restroom first.
   (B) The reunion seldom lingers, the family then retreats for the day.
   (C) The club seems merit-based until they give awards for just showing up.
   (D) When I want silence, the neighbor give me mayhem.

4. Which of the following sentences provides an example of correct subject–verb agreement?

   (A) The faculty, upon analyzing applicant records, accept only the top 100.
   (B) The team of participants is performing in orchestrated harmony.
   (C) The group of tourists, viewing the awkward map, choose the alternate path.
   (D) The crowd, pleased with the show, cheer until the band comes back.

5. When <u>Sam</u> went to visit Sally, ___ decided to take a shortcut.

   Which of the following options is the correct pronoun for the sentence above? The antecedent of the pronoun to be added is underlined.

   (A) him
   (B) she
   ✓ (C) he
   (D) her

6. While strolling with graceful Sprint and Splash, Doug and Dolly were stopped often by children wanting to pet ___ dogs.

   Which of the following is the correct pronoun to complete the sentence above?

   (A) theirs
   (B) there
   ✓ (C) their
   (D) them

7. Which of the following is an example of a correctly punctuated direct dialogue sentence?

   (A) She told me, I hope we can get together sometime again soon.
   ✓ (B) She told me, "I hope we can get together sometime again soon."
   (C) Lisa told me, "she hopes we can get together sometime again soon."
   (D) Lisa told me that "she hopes we can get together sometime again soon."

8. Which of these sentences correctly punctuates direct dialogue?

   ✓ (A) "Over any other literary style, I'd rather read poetry," confided Sandy.
   (B) I'd rather read poetry, confided Sandy, over any other literary style.
   (C) Sally confided, "I'd rather 'read poetry' over any other 'literary style.'"
   (D) Sandy confided that she'd rather read poetry over any other literary style.

9. Which of these is an example of third-person point of view?

   (A) The couple decided to leave the concert as soon as the last song started to avoid the heavy traffic.
   (B) We thought it better to leave the concert toward the start of the last song to avoid the heavy traffic.
   (C) I and my date decided to leave the concert when the last song started to avoid the heavy traffic.
   ✓ (D) You have to decide to leave the concert at the start of the last song to avoid the heavy traffic.

10. Which of these sentences in the instructions below is an example of second-person voice?

   ✓ (A) Once anyone sees the curve, it is easy to make the right and quick left turns.
   (B) After we saw the curve, we failed to see the way to turn right and then left.
   (C) As soon as you see the curve, make a right and then a quick left turn.
   (D) As soon as I missed the curve, there was no way to turn right and then left.

11. Jake and Sue worked on a project. The electric power failed. He started an electricity-free project. She called the electric company.

Which of these options best uses grammar for style and clarity to combine the sentences above?

(A) Jake and Sue worked on a project when the electric power failed; he started an electricity-free project, and she called the electric company.

(B) While Jake and Sue worked on a project, the electric power failed; he started an electricity-free project while she called the electric company.

(C) The electric power failed while Jake and Sue worked on a project; he started an electricity-free project, but she called the electric company.

(D) The electric power failed while they worked on a project; Sue called the electric company while Jake started an electricity-free project.

12. We went to the beach. The sun was warm. The water was cold. We did not swim.

Which of these options best uses grammar for style and clarity to combine the sentences above?

(A) We went to the beach, the sun was warm and the water was cold, so we did not swim.

(B) When we went to the beach, the sun was warm; however, since the water was cold, we did not swim.

(C) When we went to the beach, the sun was warm; since the water was cold, we did not swim.

(D) The sun was warm when we went to the beach, but we did not swim because the water was cold.

13. Although given at sundry times, they ignored the frequent warnings.

Which of these is the meaning of the word *sundry* as used in the sentence above?

(A) overexposed and barren
(B) several and diverse
(C) sudden and unplanned
(D) limited and common

14. Even when she said, "Don't get me wrong," she sounded supercilious.

Which of these best reflects the meaning of the word *supercilious*?

(A) humble
(B) laborious
(C) arrogant
(D) superficial

15. The physician asked if the patient's problem was related to the myotenderness.

    In the sentence above, the prefix *myo-* indicates that the physician was referring to what type of problem?

    (A) skin layer
    (B) muscle tissue
    (C) gland tissue
    (D) lung tissue

16. The politician argued from the stand of a supranational.

    In the sentence above, the prefix *supra-* can best be defined by which of these words?

    (A) below
    (B) before
    (C) beyond
    (D) beneath

17. Which of these words is spelled correctly?

    (A) Ecception
    (B) Correxion
    (C) Biseps
    (D) Acceptable

18. Which of these words is spelled correctly?

    (A) Zoologecal
    (B) Yearnin
    (C) Wicket
    (D) Virulose

19. Only after he had the _____, his work was considered finished.

    Which of these options correctly completes the sentence above?

    (A) complement
    (B) compliment
    (C) deficit
    (D) deafcet

20. _____ the one _____ shoes these are?

    Which of these options correctly complete the question above?

    (A) whom; whose
    (B) whose; whom
    (C) who's; whose
    (D) whose; who's

21. He was bemused when she said that she lived by the <u>cemetary</u>.

    Which of these words corrects the spelling of the underlined word to the sentence above?

    (A) Ceminary
    (B) Cementary
    (C) Cemetery
    (D) Cemitary

22. Which of these underlined words is an example of correct spelling?

    (A) Because her hair took longer in <u>dying</u>, her beautician kept her longer.
    (B) Her unconventional <u>genre</u> of novel writing was puzzling.
    (C) Because of the <u>stationery</u> nature of the road, he arrived late to the meeting.
    (D) Unlike your usual tardiness, <u>your</u> here early today.

23. Which of these sentences follows the rules of capitalization?

    (A) I like the month of june.
    (B) I am with Uncle Pete.
    (C) I am from The Old South.
    (D) I'll be back in Spring.

24. When we visit the city of Austin, Texas, we'd like to go to the capitol and a music event, such as the state Fair of Texas.

    Which of these words in the sentence above should be capitalized?

    (A) city
    (B) capitol
    (C) state
    (D) music

25. Which of these sentences correctly applies the rules of punctuation?

    (A) We promised to arrive on time, however; the rain kept us from keeping our promise.
    (B) We promised to arrive on time; however, the rain kept us from keeping our promise.
    (C) We promised to arrive on time, however, the rain kept us from keeping our promise.
    (D) We promised to arrive on time; however the rain kept us from keeping our promise.

26. I tried to finish the project last night but the computer broke down; instead, I did the following __ watched some television, read some book chapters, and went to bed early.

    Which of these punctuation marks correctly completes the sentence above?

    (A) ...
    (B) ,
    (C) ;
    (D) :

27. Which of these is an example of a simple sentence?

    (A) The man who waited long.
    (B) Missed lunch.
    (C) The man who was late, waited long, and missed lunch.
    (D) The man waited long, was late and missed lunch.

28. Which of these is an example of a simple sentence?

    (A) The parrot of the beautiful blue stripes had screeched for an hour but started talking with a fresh piece of apple.
    (B) The parrot of the beautiful blue stripes had screeched for an hour, but he started talking when I gave him a fresh piece of apple.
    (C) The parrot of the beautiful blue stripes had screeched for an hour until I gave him a fresh piece of apple.
    (D) The parrot of the beautiful blue stripes had screeched for an hour, although I gave him a fresh piece of apple.

29. The tourist gazed through the shopping mall. She was amazed at the countless bargains on display.

    Which of these answers uses a conjunction to combine the sentences above so that the focus is more on the tourist's amazement and less on her gazing through the mall?

    (A) The tourist gazed through the shopping mall; she was amazed at the countless bargains on display.
    (B) The tourist gazed through the shopping mall and was amazed at the countless bargains on display.
    (C) As the tourist gazed through the shopping mall, she was amazed at the countless bargains on display.
    (D) The tourist gazed through the shopping mall, and she was amazed at the countless bargains on display.

30. The student who makes the highest grades _____

    Which of these allows the above sentence to be completed as a simple sentence?

    (A) sits mid-classroom and often offers help.
    (B) sits mid-classroom, and some have often used his help.
    (C) gets along well, although some think him odd.
    (D) gets along well after we had him included in our team.

31. Which of these sentences is most clear and correct?

    (A) When the sun was just about to set the climbers made it to the zenith.
    (B) The climbers made it to the zenith when the sun was just about to set.
    (C) The climbers reached the zenith near sunset.
    (D) About sunset, the climbers made it to the zenith.

32. We went to town. The machine broke. The mechanic said it was a wheeling piece. We bought it new.

To improve sentence fluency, which of these best states the information above in a single sentence?

(A) When we went to town, the machine broke and the mechanic said it was a wheeling piece, so we bought it new.

(B) When we went to town and the machine broke, the mechanic said it was a wheeling piece, then we bought it new.

(C) When the machine broke and the mechanic said it was a wheeling piece, we went to town and bought it new.

(D) When the machine broke, and the mechanic said it was a wheeling piece, we bought it new when we went to town.

33. I started reading a book. I could not put it down. I spent the whole night up. I overslept.

To improve sentence fluency, which of these best states the information above in a single sentence?

(A) I started reading a book and I could not put it down, so I spent the whole night up and I overslept.

(B) I started reading a book, but I could not put it down, so I spent the whole night up, and overslept.

(C) I spent the whole night up and I overslept because I started reading a book, and I could not put it down.

(D) I overslept because I spent the whole night up, since I started reading a book, and I could not put it down.

34. We went to the backfield. The dogs came along. We had a great time. We returned at dusk.

To improve sentence fluency, which of these best states the information above in a single sentence?

(A) We went to the backfield, and the dogs came along, we had a great time, so we returned at dusk.

(B) We went to the backfield and the dogs came along, we returned at dusk because we had a great time.

(C) When we went to the backfield the dogs came along, and we had a great time as we returned at dusk.

(D) The dogs came along when we went to the backfield and, because we had a great time, we returned at dusk.

ANSWER KEY
Practice Test 1

READING

1.	C	13.	A	25.	A	37.	D
2.	B	14.	B	26.	C	38.	B
3.	A	15.	B	27.	C	39.	D
4.	A	16.	D	28.	B	40.	A
5.	D	17.	C	29.	C	41.	C
6.	D	18.	D	30.	D	42.	A
7.	C	19.	A	31.	B	43.	D
8.	A	20.	A	32.	C	44.	D
9.	B	21.	C	33.	B	45.	A
10.	D	22.	A	34.	C	46.	B
11.	B	23.	C	35.	B	47.	B
12.	C	24.	D	36.	B	48.	C

MATHEMATICS

1.	D	10.	D	19.	B	28.	C
2.	B	11.	B	20.	D	29.	A
3.	C	12.	D	21.	D	30.	D
4.	C	13.	C	22.	B	31.	A
5.	B	14.	A	23.	B	32.	C
6.	D	15.	D	24.	D	33.	B
7.	C	16.	B	25.	D	34.	C
8.	A	17.	A	26.	A		
9.	B	18.	C	27.	C		

SCIENCE

1.	C	**15.**	A	**29.**	B	**43.**	D
2.	D	**16.**	C	**30.**	C	**44.**	C
3.	B	**17.**	A	**31.**	D	**45.**	A
4.	A	**18.**	B	**32.**	B	**46.**	B
5.	B	**19.**	A	**33.**	A	**47.**	C
6.	A	**20.**	C	**34.**	D	**48.**	D
7.	C	**21.**	C	**35.**	A	**49.**	B
8.	B	**22.**	B	**36.**	B	**50.**	A
9.	D	**23.**	D	**37.**	D	**51.**	B
10.	C	**24.**	A	**38.**	C	**52.**	C
11.	B	**25.**	B	**39.**	A	**53.**	A
12.	B	**26.**	C	**40.**	B	**54.**	D
13.	D	**27.**	B	**41.**	D		
14.	D	**28.**	D	**42.**	A		

ENGLISH AND LANGUAGE USAGE

1.	D	**10.**	C	**19.**	A	**28.**	B
2.	C	**11.**	C	**20.**	C	**29.**	C
3.	B	**12.**	D	**21.**	C	**30.**	A
4.	B	**13.**	B	**22.**	B	**31.**	B
5.	C	**14.**	C	**23.**	B	**32.**	D
6.	C	**15.**	B	**24.**	C	**33.**	C
7.	B	**16.**	C	**25.**	B	**34.**	D
8.	A	**17.**	D	**26.**	D		
9.	A	**18.**	C	**27.**	C		

ANSWER EXPLANATIONS
Reading

1. **(C)** The title represents a detail. The theme and topic could be considered the view of each partner in the relationship. The main idea is interpretation of love as defined by each person in the story.

2. **(B)** Narrative style tells a story. Expository passages explain a topic or subject in order to increase understanding of ideas. Technical writing usually addresses precise information. Persuasive writing tries to convince the reader to agree with the author.

3. **(A)** This is the general idea expressed by the author. The other choices reflect more specific statements, supporting details, or an overused expression applied incorrectly.

4. **(A)** This was intended to entertain the reader similar to most fiction passages. Poetry is often used to evoke emotions. This passage was not intended to delineate a universal fact or to persuade the reader toward a judgment.

5. **(D)** The passage describes an event or person. A sequence is usually expressed as a bulleted or numbered list. A comparison-contrast structure has two opposing ideas that force the reader to identify differences. The cause and effect would describe an event with expected consequences.

6. **(D)** This response best describes the character's overall belief about the events. The other responses reflect actual statements from the passage.

7. **(C)** This passage was intended to describe a particular medical practice. Poetry is often used to evoke emotions. Fiction entertains the reader. The author was not trying to persuade the reader about a particular practice of health care.

8. **(A)** The author was explaining a topic or subject in order to increase understanding of ideas or using expository writing. Technical writing usually addresses precise information. Persuasive writing tries to convince the reader to agree with the author. Narrative style tells a story.

9. **(B)** The theory was developed over 4000 years ago. Web site information could be a primary source but could also be inaccurate. There is no evidence that the passage was based on a primary source.

10. **(D)** The passage describes a cultural difference in health care. A sequence is usually expressed as a bulleted or numbered list. A comparison-contrast structure has two opposing ideas that force the reader to identify a difference. The cause and effect would describe an event with expected consequences.

11. **(B)** This is a supporting detail expressed by the author. The statement is too specific to be an overall topic, main idea, or theme.

12. **(C)** The overall intent of the passage is to express the author's opinion on the balance of benefit to expense on attending a workshop. The other answers do not mention an overall experience but are focused on specific experiences or express emotions and feelings opposite to the statements in the passage.

13. **(A)** The passage seems to be from the business section of a newspaper. The author was not trying to persuade you to purchase something or trying to get you to laugh. Most business articles provide straightforward information.

14. **(B)** The passage is an advertisement and is selling a product. This passage was to persuade the reader to make the purchase.

15. **(B)** This article summarizes the flux of stock market and the current economy. The only concrete statement was in the section about the influence of the Federal Reserve on bonds. The rest of the passage suggests a variable unpredictable market. The last response is in opposition to the overall message.

16. **(D)** The overall purpose is for the reader to contrast-compare the different legislative actions between times of plenty and deficit.

17. **(C)** A political ad is always considered to be a way to persuade you to vote for one candidate instead of another.

18. **(D)** This passage is a narrative. A narrative or storytelling passage is usually done to entertain. One thing leads to another in a chain of causal events.

19. **(A)** This is most likely taken from a textbook since it is informative in nature. It is not written to entertain so it is not from a novel. It is not written with a technical focus so it is not likely from a research journal.

20. **(A)** The email is definitely written to convince the HR Director that Mary should be hired.

21. **(C)** The author has a bias toward Mary being hired and is open about it.

22. **(A)** The article is about women's fashion and the openings in the fabric of the formal dresses worn at the festival.

23. **(C)** FALLING
    FIALLNG
    FILLNG
    FILNG
    FIL
    FILE

24. **(D)** Making Paths and Walkways 108

25. **(A)** May 21

26. **(C)** 7 years

27. **(C)** Chicken costs at least $0.30 less than the other meat and fish.

28. **(B)** 4946

29. **(C)**

30. **(D)** Milk chocolate is the correct response: it is a combination of cocoa and milk. Soy milk is a synthetic that does not contain any animal protein.

31. **(B)** Fiber 11 Grams

32. **(C)** A popular travel handbook for the Islands of Northern Europe published in 2011. This would provide current information that would be unbiased.

33. **(B)** labor

34. **(C)** 10

35. **(B)** more than 5 pounds less than 10 pounds (7.5 pounds)

36. **(B)** 20°

37. **(D)** 1, the family will pass refreshments when they travel between Re and Fo.

38. **(B)** Point #2 Topic Sentence

39. **(D)** Example

40. **(A)** candidatestance.org, all candidate review

41. **(C)** to identify who is involved in the dialogue

42. **(A)** to denote the beginning and end of a statement

43. **(D)** the area has a thirty percent chance of receiving some rainfall

44. **(D)** motorcycles

45. **(A)** persuade

46. **(B)** Lenox, MA

47. **(B)** Asia. The other responses are very specific regions, rather than general as the outline suggests.

48. **(C)** 5 Related Information

Mathematics

1. **(D)** $40+(4\times(5+3)^2) =$

    $40+(4\times 64)\quad =$

    $40+256\qquad\quad = 296$

Simplify the expression with the innermost parentheses first, after clearing the exponent. Then solve the equation in the next parentheses: 40 + 256 = 296

2. **(B)** 0.114 − 32.22 =

    −32.220
    +00.114
    −32.106

With regroup activity

```
       1
 -32.2 2 ¹0
 +00.1 1 4
 -32.1 0 6
```

Arrange the numbers in rows with decimals aligned and the larger number at the top. Match decimal places by adding 0 to match the column length for each number. Begin subtraction from the far right column by carrying forward of tenths, ones, and tens as indicated to regroup for whole number computation.

3. **(C)** $10.00 - ((5 \times 0.29) + (9 \times 0.44)) =$

$10.00 - (1.45 + 3.96) \qquad =$

$10.00 - 5.41 \qquad\qquad = \$4.59$

Solve in each parentheses first. Then subtract from the overall payment to determine the change to be returned.

4. **(C)** $3\dfrac{1}{2} = \dfrac{7}{2},$

$6\dfrac{1}{3} = \dfrac{19}{3},$

$\dfrac{7}{2} \times \dfrac{3}{3} = \dfrac{21}{6},$

$\dfrac{19}{3} \times \dfrac{2}{2} = \dfrac{38}{6},$

$\dfrac{(21+38)}{6} = \dfrac{59}{6} = 9\dfrac{5}{6}$

Convert to an improper fraction. Find the least common denominator (number under the line in the fraction).

Add the numerators (numbers above the line in the fraction).

Convert the improper fraction to a simplified fraction.

5. **(B)** What is the product of the numbers 0.45 × 1/6?

$$
\begin{array}{r}
0.166 \\
\times 0.45 \\
\hline
830 \\
664 \quad \\
\hline
0.07470
\end{array}
$$

0.075

Convert the fraction to a decimal by dividing the numerator by the denominator. Complete the computation and then count the decimal spaces to count from the right for the correct places. Round up to simplify.

6. **(D)** 9 divided by $\dfrac{1}{4} =$

$9 \times \dfrac{4}{1} = 36$

When dividing by a fraction the reciprocal (inverted fraction) is used to multiply.

7. **(C)** $\dfrac{15}{1}$ as $\dfrac{128}{x} =$

$15x = 128$

$\dfrac{15x}{15} = \dfrac{128}{15}$

$\dfrac{128}{15} = 8.53$

Cross multiply (the numerator of the first number is multiplied by the denominator of the second number) and divide. Then round up to the nearest whole number since a person cannot be divided into parts and the ratio cannot be increased.

8. **(A)** $5 \times 60 = 300$ minutes

$$\frac{30}{300} = \frac{1}{10}$$

Convert hours to minutes. Then write ratio numbers in a fraction. Simplify the fraction. There are ten 30-minute segments in 5 hours.

9. **(B)** 0.125 divided by 0.2

$$
\begin{array}{r}
0.625 \\
2\overline{)1.250} \\
\underline{12} \\
5 \\
\underline{4} \\
10 \\
\underline{10} \\
0
\end{array}
$$

Remove decimals from divisor (0.2) by moving the decimal to the right. Then move the equivalent numbers of decimal points in the dividend (0.125). Match decimal location on line above dividend and divide.

10. **(D)** $\left(\sqrt{10}\right)$ Think about the closest square root to this number and that will be the answer.

11. **(B)** 8% = 0.08 in decimal

$$\frac{12{,}100}{0.08}$$

$$.08\overline{)12100.00}$$

$$
\begin{array}{r}
151250 \\
8\overline{)1210000} \\
\underline{8} \\
41 \\
\underline{40} \\
10 \\
\underline{8} \\
20 \\
\underline{16} \\
40 \\
\underline{40} \\
0
\end{array}
$$

Convert the percent to a decimal and divide by the decimal obtained.

12. **(D)** Divide 1 by 32 = 0.03. Count two decimal spaces to the right and place the % sign after the whole number.

13. **(C)** Convert 33% to a fraction. Place the percent over 100 and simplify the fraction.

14. **(A)** $\dfrac{1{,}000 - 890}{1{,}000} = 11$ percent decrease in enrollment

15. **(D)** Convert each fraction to a common denominator and then rank by largest numerator. A $\frac{234}{300}$, B $\frac{200}{300}$, C $\frac{150}{300}$, D $\frac{250}{300}$

16. **(B)** Since this is an estimate, start with the easiest numbers to multiply. Try C: $20 \times 30 = 600$. Next try A: $30 \times 30 = 900$ is too high, so you know the answer is B.

17. **(A)** $(4250 + 680 + 420) - (1100 + 350) =$
$$5350 - 1450 = \$3900$$

18. **(C)** $4125 \times .25 = 1031.25$

19. **(B)** $800 \times 1.02 = \$816 \times 52$ weeks $= \$42,432$

20. **(D)** 1974

    M = 1000, C = 100, L = 50, X = 10, V = 5. I = 1. If a smaller number is listed before M, L, X, or V, it will be subtracted from the main number. Traditionally the numbers that follow in decreasing order add to the total number.

    M = 1000, CM = 900 (1000 − 100), LXX = 70 (50 + 20), IV = 4 (5 − 1)

21. **(D)** 1 kilometer = 0.62 miles, $4 \times 0.62 = 2.48$

22. **(B)** $3.785 \times 2 = 7.570$ liters

23. **(B)** 1 pound = 0.45 kilograms, 1 ounce = 28 grams. The child lost 8 oz $\times$ 28 = 224 grams.

24. **(D)** prefix centi $= \frac{1}{100}$ of a meter.

25. **(D)** milliliter

26. **(A)** $150 \times 6.5 = 975$

27. **(C)** A dependent variable is dependent upon the changes being implemented in research.

28. **(C)** The total of the two sections of concern is 39%. $(2000 \times 0.39 = 780)$

29. **(A)** A pie chart is designed to accommodate all characteristics of concern such as demographics or characteristics of a community. A bar graph provides a way to compare higher/lower or change in data over time. A Gantt chart enables a researcher to plan the project with specific dates and benchmarks. A histogram demonstrates a distribution around a mean.

30. **(D)** $\dfrac{(12xy + 8xy^2 - 4xy)}{24xy}$

    $\dfrac{8xy^2 - 4xy + 12xy}{24xy}$

    $\dfrac{8xy^2 + 8xy}{24xy}$

    $\dfrac{y+1}{3}$

    $\dfrac{1}{3}y + \dfrac{1}{3}$

31. **(A)** The father's age x is equal to 3 times the daughter's age y plus 5.

32. **(C)** $\dfrac{x}{2}+5=9$

$\dfrac{x}{2}+5-5=9-5$

$\dfrac{x}{2}=4$

$\dfrac{x(2)}{21}=4(2)=8$

33. **(B)** Solve this equation for j: $j + 3 = 7$

$j+3(-3)=7(-3)$

$j=4$

34. **(C)** $[x-20]>5$

$x<15$ or $x>25$

Since there is a lesser than number the connector will be 'or'
Solve the problem without the absolute number sign.
$x - 20 > 5$, > becomes + then $x > 25$
$x - 20 < 5$, < becomes – then $x < 15$.

Science

1. **(C)** The number of protons is equal to the atomic number located on the periodic chart. Magnesium (Mg) has 12.

2. **(D)** 28 The number of neutrons = Atomic mass – Atomic number

3. **(B)** Potential energy is stored energy. As the amusement ride is not moving on its own, energy is being stored. Kinetic energy is the energy of motion.

4. **(A)** The number of electrons if the atom is neutral must have enough negative charges to offset the proton's positive charge. It will be 8 since that is the number of protons.

5. **(B)** A catalyst in a chemical reaction controls the rate of the reaction.

6. **(A)** Metals will conduct electricity and also heat and cool rapidly.

7. **(C)** Covalent bonds share electrons.

8. **(B)** This is an electron attraction.

9. **(D)** Acid and base solutions when combined will release an ionic neutral salt.

10. **(C)** The formula is H = M × L H 200 grams × 540 calories = 108,000 = 108 kilocalories.

11. **(B)** Inductive reasoning is taking a specific idea and moving it to a global perspective.

12. **(B)** This quantitative study should demonstrate random selection, random assignment to experimental and control groups, and then evaluation after the group specific intervention. Of course, the researcher can then cross over to allow the control group to have a chance.

13. **(D)** Randomly divide study participants into groups, measure the severity of headache pain before providing the same foods to one group, provide a placebo to the other group, and then measure the severity of headaches one hour after the food or placebo was given.

14. **(D)** Formulating the question would follow problem identification.

15. **(A)** Repeated testing over time with the same results increases confidence in a theory.

16. **(C)** Technology and mathematics assist in describing relationships between data sets.

17. **(A)** The upward slope of the line in the graph suggests that as the vehicle increases in weight there is more pressure on tires.

18. **(B)** The line shows an increase in one measurement when the other is increasing; this is a direct relationship.

19. **(A)** Research should be used in life, so this would suggest that tire inflation checks are important when varying the load of a vehicle.

20. **(C)** Dependent variables will need an action influencing (independent) the activity.

21. **(C)** As the variable increased the results increased. This is a direct relationship.

22. **(B)** Repeating the study would be a waste of time since all of the studies revealed the same results. The researcher could try to establish a minimum effective disinfectant level.

23. **(D)** Part of the scientific method is to investigate the problem then to identify the problem.

24. **(A)** The end of a scientific report on research data should include a conclusion or discussion at the end. The rest of these steps would have been completed before the discussion phase.

25. **(B)** The endocrine system regulates the internal environment of the mammalian body.

26. **(C)** The dorsal body area contains the brain and spinal cord. The spleen occupies the ventral body cavity with the rest of the abdominal organs.

27. **(B)** The finger would be distal to any other structure on the hand or forearm.

28. **(D)** Deoxygenated blood enters the heart from the structure accepting all venous blood from the rest of the body, the right atrium.

29. **(B)** Oxygenated blood enters the heart from the pulmonary veins into the left atrium, mitral valve, left ventricle and then is pumped to the rest of the body.

30. **(C)** During expiration carbon dioxide leaves the lungs.

31. **(D)** The alveoli begin the internal respiratory process.

32. **(B)** Proteins are digested primarily in the stomach. The digestion of protein is essential for the production of the intrinsic factor that occurs in the stomach.

33. **(A)** The villi in the small intestine increase the surface area of the structure and thus the ability to absorb nutrients.

34. **(D)** The skin is the body's first defense against invasion by bacteria and viruses.

35. **(A)** Active immunity is acquired from direct exposure to a pathogen.

36. **(B)** The nervous system is considered to be the controller of the organism.

37. **(D)** The respiratory and urinary systems are involved in acid base balance and the body's buffer system.

38. **(C)** Underdeveloped countries will have as high as seven children per woman. More developed countries will have as few as one child per woman.

39. **(A)** Overpopulation occurs when the crude birth rate exceeds crude death rate.

40. **(B)** Enzymes are used primarily in the digestive processes.

41. **(D)** The gall bladder produces bile for fat digestion.

42. **(A)** Immigration is a major factor influencing population growth.

43. **(D)** DNA carries the genetic structure of each cell.

44. **(C)** Adaptation is a change in genetic composition of an organism over time such as antibiotic resistance.

45. **(A)** Thymine is found in DNA but not in RNA.

46. **(B)** Prokaryotic cells do not have a nucleus.

47. **(C)** Chloroplasts are in plant cells and produce plant energy called chlorophyll.

48. **(D)** G_1, RNA pairing with their DNA partner, then the S phase begins.

49. **(B)** Reproductive cells use the process of meiosis as cell replication, producing four separate cells at a division.

50. **(A)** Cells require mitochondria for respiration.

51. **(B)** The genetic traits of the cells are contained in the proteins in DNA and RNA.

52. **(C)** Germ cells are the only cells that can alter the organism with mutations across generations.

53. **(A)** Phenotypes determine the code for skin and hair color and other inherited traits.

54. **(D)** To answer this type of genetic question, draw a Punnett square to determine the percentage of traits in each organism. (**tt** are seedless and **Tt** have seeds). The offspring will have a 50% chance of providing seedless grapes.

	T	**t**
t	Tt	tt
t	Tt	tt

English and Language Usage

1. **(D)** This option contains the proper adverb *suddenly* to complete the sentence. The other options are incorrect in either grammar or case.

2. **(C)** This option correctly identifies *receiving* as a verb and *reluctantly* as an adverb.

3. **(B)** This option contains correct subject–verb agreement: "reunion… lingers" and "family… retreats." All other options contain incorrect subject–verb agreement with regard to number.

4. **(B)** This option contains correct subject–verb agreement: "the team… is." All other options contain incorrect subject–verb agreement with regard to number.

5. **(C)** The antecedent, *Sam*, is singular and masculine, which means that *he* is the only correct answer. All other options are incorrect either in number, gender, or case.

6. **(C)** This option correctly completes the sentence as it contains the correct pronoun to use. All other options are incorrect pronouns to use in this case.

7. **(B)** This option correctly contains double quotation marks around the whole quote. Option A has no quotation marks to properly indicate direct dialogue, and options B and D contain quotations in the wrong places.

8. **(A)** This option correctly contains double quotation marks around the whole quote. Option B has no quotation marks to properly indicate direct dialogue, option C contains quotations in the wrong places, and option D unnecessarily adds single quotes.

9. **(A)** This option is an example of third-person point of view. Options B and C are examples of first-person point of view. Option D is an example of second-person point of view.

10. **(C)** This option is an example of second-person point of view. Options B and D are examples of first-person point of view. Option A is an example of third-person point of view.

11. **(C)** This option effectively uses transitional words to combine the sentences into a single sentence to reflect the original meaning of the group of sentences. All other options may lead to confusion of the writer's original intent.

12. **(D)** This option effectively uses transitional words to combine the sentences into a single sentence that still reflects the original meaning of the group of sentences.

13. **(B)** This option rightly and properly defines the word *sundry* (which has nothing to do with *sun-dried*). All other options are incorrect.

14. **(C)** This option correctly defines the word *supercilious*. All other options are incorrect.

15. **(B)** The prefix *myo-* originates from the Greek language. The word *myotenderness* means "muscular tenderness." Therefore, it can be concluded that this physician was referring to a condition related to muscular pain or discomfort.

16. **(C)** The prefix *supra-* originates from the Latin language. The word *supranational* means "beyond or outside the jurisdiction of any nation." Therefore, it can be concluded that this politician was not interested in local politics.

17. **(D)** This option is the correct spelling: *acceptable* is a commonly misspelled word; it has two *c*'s and ends in *le*.

18. **(C)** This option alone is spelled correctly. All other options are spelled incorrectly.

19. **(A)** This option contains the correct word that completes the given sentence. The sentence ending in "considered finished" adds strength to the meaning of *complement*.

20. **(C)** This option contains the only word-set that completes the given sentence. *Who's* and *whose* are commonly misspelled homophone (sound alike) words.

21. **(C)** This option is spelled correctly: *cemetery* is a commonly misspelled word; it has three *e*'s and ends in *y*. The verb *bemused* (puzzled or baffled) offers a cue to identify *cemetery* as the correctly spelled word.

22. **(B)** This option is spelled correctly. All other options are commonly misspelled words: *dying* (about to die) is not *dyeing* (coloring), *stationery* (desk items) is not *stationary* (unmoving, as in bad traffic), and *your* (possessive pronoun) is not *you're* (contraction of *you are*).

23. **(B)** The word *Uncle* is properly capitalized, as it does not follow the possessive *my*. None of the other options follow correct rules of capitalization.

24. **(C)** The word *state* should be capitalized, as it is used as a proper noun in this context. There is no need to capitalize the words in options A, B, or D.

25. **(B)** This option is correctly punctuated with the conjunctive adverb preceded by a semicolon and followed by a comma.

26. **(D)** To correctly punctuate the sentence, a semicolon is required to precede the conjunctive adverbs that connect sentence elements of equal rank, as in *however* in this case.

27. **(C)** This option is constructed as a simple sentence containing one subject and one verb. Although the sentence is detailed, there are no clauses adding to the complexity of the sentence structure, as is the case in option D. Options A and B are not complete sentences.

28. **(B)** This option is constructed as a simple sentence with one subject and a compound verb. Although the sentence is detailed, there are no clauses adding to the complexity of the sentence structure, as in the case of all other options.

29. **(C)** This option makes one clause subordinate to the other by the addition of a subordinating conjunction. All other options contain two clauses of equal weight.

30. **(A)** This option completes the sentence as a simple sentence. All other options are examples of compound sentences.

31. **(B)** This option clearly and succinctly conveys the writer's intent to accurately describe the event. The other options are written in ways in which the writer's intent might be confused.

32. **(D)** This option is an example of the use of grammar to enhance clarity and readability. The four sentences are combined into one clear, succinct sentence that is easy to read and understand. The other options, while employing correct grammar to condense the four sentences, do not do so in a manner that clearly expresses the writer's intent.

33. **(C)** This option effectively uses transitional words to combine the sentences into a single sentence that still reflects the original meaning of the group of sentences.

34. **(D)** This option effectively uses transitional words to combine the sentences into a single sentence that still reflects the original meaning of the group of sentences.

Practice
TEST 2

ANSWER SHEET
Practice Test 2

READING

1. Ⓐ Ⓑ Ⓒ Ⓓ	13. Ⓐ Ⓑ Ⓒ Ⓓ	25. Ⓐ Ⓑ Ⓒ Ⓓ	37. Ⓐ Ⓑ Ⓒ Ⓓ
2. Ⓐ Ⓑ Ⓒ Ⓓ	14. Ⓐ Ⓑ Ⓒ Ⓓ	26. Ⓐ Ⓑ Ⓒ Ⓓ	38. Ⓐ Ⓑ Ⓒ Ⓓ
3. Ⓐ Ⓑ Ⓒ Ⓓ	15. Ⓐ Ⓑ Ⓒ Ⓓ	27. Ⓐ Ⓑ Ⓒ Ⓓ	39. Ⓐ Ⓑ Ⓒ Ⓓ
4. Ⓐ Ⓑ Ⓒ Ⓓ	16. Ⓐ Ⓑ Ⓒ Ⓓ	28. Ⓐ Ⓑ Ⓒ Ⓓ	40. Ⓐ Ⓑ Ⓒ Ⓓ
5. Ⓐ Ⓑ Ⓒ Ⓓ	17. Ⓐ Ⓑ Ⓒ Ⓓ	29. Ⓐ Ⓑ Ⓒ Ⓓ	41. Ⓐ Ⓑ Ⓒ Ⓓ
6. Ⓐ Ⓑ Ⓒ Ⓓ	18. Ⓐ Ⓑ Ⓒ Ⓓ	30. Ⓐ Ⓑ Ⓒ Ⓓ	42. Ⓐ Ⓑ Ⓒ Ⓓ
7. Ⓐ Ⓑ Ⓒ Ⓓ	19. Ⓐ Ⓑ Ⓒ Ⓓ	31. Ⓐ Ⓑ Ⓒ Ⓓ	43. Ⓐ Ⓑ Ⓒ Ⓓ
8. Ⓐ Ⓑ Ⓒ Ⓓ	20. Ⓐ Ⓑ Ⓒ Ⓓ	32. Ⓐ Ⓑ Ⓒ Ⓓ	44. Ⓐ Ⓑ Ⓒ Ⓓ
9. Ⓐ Ⓑ Ⓒ Ⓓ	21. Ⓐ Ⓑ Ⓒ Ⓓ	33. Ⓐ Ⓑ Ⓒ Ⓓ	45. Ⓐ Ⓑ Ⓒ Ⓓ
10. Ⓐ Ⓑ Ⓒ Ⓓ	22. Ⓐ Ⓑ Ⓒ Ⓓ	34. Ⓐ Ⓑ Ⓒ Ⓓ	46. Ⓐ Ⓑ Ⓒ Ⓓ
11. Ⓐ Ⓑ Ⓒ Ⓓ	23. Ⓐ Ⓑ Ⓒ Ⓓ	35. Ⓐ Ⓑ Ⓒ Ⓓ	47. Ⓐ Ⓑ Ⓒ Ⓓ
12. Ⓐ Ⓑ Ⓒ Ⓓ	24. Ⓐ Ⓑ Ⓒ Ⓓ	36. Ⓐ Ⓑ Ⓒ Ⓓ	48. Ⓐ Ⓑ Ⓒ Ⓓ

MATHEMATICS

1. Ⓐ Ⓑ Ⓒ Ⓓ	10. Ⓐ Ⓑ Ⓒ Ⓓ	19. Ⓐ Ⓑ Ⓒ Ⓓ	28. Ⓐ Ⓑ Ⓒ Ⓓ
2. Ⓐ Ⓑ Ⓒ Ⓓ	11. Ⓐ Ⓑ Ⓒ Ⓓ	20. Ⓐ Ⓑ Ⓒ Ⓓ	29. Ⓐ Ⓑ Ⓒ Ⓓ
3. Ⓐ Ⓑ Ⓒ Ⓓ	12. Ⓐ Ⓑ Ⓒ Ⓓ	21. Ⓐ Ⓑ Ⓒ Ⓓ	30. Ⓐ Ⓑ Ⓒ Ⓓ
4. Ⓐ Ⓑ Ⓒ Ⓓ	13. Ⓐ Ⓑ Ⓒ Ⓓ	22. Ⓐ Ⓑ Ⓒ Ⓓ	31. Ⓐ Ⓑ Ⓒ Ⓓ
5. Ⓐ Ⓑ Ⓒ Ⓓ	14. Ⓐ Ⓑ Ⓒ Ⓓ	23. Ⓐ Ⓑ Ⓒ Ⓓ	32. Ⓐ Ⓑ Ⓒ Ⓓ
6. Ⓐ Ⓑ Ⓒ Ⓓ	15. Ⓐ Ⓑ Ⓒ Ⓓ	24. Ⓐ Ⓑ Ⓒ Ⓓ	33. Ⓐ Ⓑ Ⓒ Ⓓ
7. Ⓐ Ⓑ Ⓒ Ⓓ	16. Ⓐ Ⓑ Ⓒ Ⓓ	25. Ⓐ Ⓑ Ⓒ Ⓓ	34. Ⓐ Ⓑ Ⓒ Ⓓ
8. Ⓐ Ⓑ Ⓒ Ⓓ	17. Ⓐ Ⓑ Ⓒ Ⓓ	26. Ⓐ Ⓑ Ⓒ Ⓓ	
9. Ⓐ Ⓑ Ⓒ Ⓓ	18. Ⓐ Ⓑ Ⓒ Ⓓ	27. Ⓐ Ⓑ Ⓒ Ⓓ	

SCIENCE

1. Ⓐ Ⓑ Ⓒ Ⓓ
2. Ⓐ Ⓑ Ⓒ Ⓓ
3. Ⓐ Ⓑ Ⓒ Ⓓ
4. Ⓐ Ⓑ Ⓒ Ⓓ
5. Ⓐ Ⓑ Ⓒ Ⓓ
6. Ⓐ Ⓑ Ⓒ Ⓓ
7. Ⓐ Ⓑ Ⓒ Ⓓ
8. Ⓐ Ⓑ Ⓒ Ⓓ
9. Ⓐ Ⓑ Ⓒ Ⓓ
10. Ⓐ Ⓑ Ⓒ Ⓓ
11. Ⓐ Ⓑ Ⓒ Ⓓ
12. Ⓐ Ⓑ Ⓒ Ⓓ
13. Ⓐ Ⓑ Ⓒ Ⓓ
14. Ⓐ Ⓑ Ⓒ Ⓓ

15. Ⓐ Ⓑ Ⓒ Ⓓ
16. Ⓐ Ⓑ Ⓒ Ⓓ
17. Ⓐ Ⓑ Ⓒ Ⓓ
18. Ⓐ Ⓑ Ⓒ Ⓓ
19. Ⓐ Ⓑ Ⓒ Ⓓ
20. Ⓐ Ⓑ Ⓒ Ⓓ
21. Ⓐ Ⓑ Ⓒ Ⓓ
22. Ⓐ Ⓑ Ⓒ Ⓓ
23. Ⓐ Ⓑ Ⓒ Ⓓ
24. Ⓐ Ⓑ Ⓒ Ⓓ
25. Ⓐ Ⓑ Ⓒ Ⓓ
26. Ⓐ Ⓑ Ⓒ Ⓓ
27. Ⓐ Ⓑ Ⓒ Ⓓ
28. Ⓐ Ⓑ Ⓒ Ⓓ

29. Ⓐ Ⓑ Ⓒ Ⓓ
30. Ⓐ Ⓑ Ⓒ Ⓓ
31. Ⓐ Ⓑ Ⓒ Ⓓ
32. Ⓐ Ⓑ Ⓒ Ⓓ
33. Ⓐ Ⓑ Ⓒ Ⓓ
34. Ⓐ Ⓑ Ⓒ Ⓓ
35. Ⓐ Ⓑ Ⓒ Ⓓ
36. Ⓐ Ⓑ Ⓒ Ⓓ
37. Ⓐ Ⓑ Ⓒ Ⓓ
38. Ⓐ Ⓑ Ⓒ Ⓓ
39. Ⓐ Ⓑ Ⓒ Ⓓ
40. Ⓐ Ⓑ Ⓒ Ⓓ
41. Ⓐ Ⓑ Ⓒ Ⓓ
42. Ⓐ Ⓑ Ⓒ Ⓓ

43. Ⓐ Ⓑ Ⓒ Ⓓ
44. Ⓐ Ⓑ Ⓒ Ⓓ
45. Ⓐ Ⓑ Ⓒ Ⓓ
46. Ⓐ Ⓑ Ⓒ Ⓓ
47. Ⓐ Ⓑ Ⓒ Ⓓ
48. Ⓐ Ⓑ Ⓒ Ⓓ
49. Ⓐ Ⓑ Ⓒ Ⓓ
50. Ⓐ Ⓑ Ⓒ Ⓓ
51. Ⓐ Ⓑ Ⓒ Ⓓ
52. Ⓐ Ⓑ Ⓒ Ⓓ
53. Ⓐ Ⓑ Ⓒ Ⓓ
54. Ⓐ Ⓑ Ⓒ Ⓓ

ENGLISH AND LANGUAGE USAGE

1. Ⓐ Ⓑ Ⓒ Ⓓ
2. Ⓐ Ⓑ Ⓒ Ⓓ
3. Ⓐ Ⓑ Ⓒ Ⓓ
4. Ⓐ Ⓑ Ⓒ Ⓓ
5. Ⓐ Ⓑ Ⓒ Ⓓ
6. Ⓐ Ⓑ Ⓒ Ⓓ
7. Ⓐ Ⓑ Ⓒ Ⓓ
8. Ⓐ Ⓑ Ⓒ Ⓓ
9. Ⓐ Ⓑ Ⓒ Ⓓ

10. Ⓐ Ⓑ Ⓒ Ⓓ
11. Ⓐ Ⓑ Ⓒ Ⓓ
12. Ⓐ Ⓑ Ⓒ Ⓓ
13. Ⓐ Ⓑ Ⓒ Ⓓ
14. Ⓐ Ⓑ Ⓒ Ⓓ
15. Ⓐ Ⓑ Ⓒ Ⓓ
16. Ⓐ Ⓑ Ⓒ Ⓓ
17. Ⓐ Ⓑ Ⓒ Ⓓ
18. Ⓐ Ⓑ Ⓒ Ⓓ

19. Ⓐ Ⓑ Ⓒ Ⓓ
20. Ⓐ Ⓑ Ⓒ Ⓓ
21. Ⓐ Ⓑ Ⓒ Ⓓ
22. Ⓐ Ⓑ Ⓒ Ⓓ
23. Ⓐ Ⓑ Ⓒ Ⓓ
24. Ⓐ Ⓑ Ⓒ Ⓓ
25. Ⓐ Ⓑ Ⓒ Ⓓ
26. Ⓐ Ⓑ Ⓒ Ⓓ
27. Ⓐ Ⓑ Ⓒ Ⓓ

28. Ⓐ Ⓑ Ⓒ Ⓓ
29. Ⓐ Ⓑ Ⓒ Ⓓ
30. Ⓐ Ⓑ Ⓒ Ⓓ
31. Ⓐ Ⓑ Ⓒ Ⓓ
32. Ⓐ Ⓑ Ⓒ Ⓓ
33. Ⓐ Ⓑ Ⓒ Ⓓ
34. Ⓐ Ⓑ Ⓒ Ⓓ

Part 1: Reading

Time: 58 minutes

48 questions

QUESTIONS 1 THROUGH 6 ARE BASED ON THE FOLLOWING PASSAGE.

The Marathon

It is common knowledge that all true athletes train in advance for competition. Mary was attracted to Mark. Mark is an excellent runner and trained by running six miles a day with adequate hydration and carbohydrate loading. Mary wanted to develop a common interest with Mark to make their relationship closer. She signed up for the same five-kilometer race as Mark. Her approach to training was different than Mark's. She measured the exact distance from her home to run exactly three miles three days per week.

She was definitely excited about the race and told her friends about her plans at a party the night before the event. Mary's group wanted to really help her decrease her anxiety about performance so they stayed late to talk to her about how great she was training.

The morning of the marathon, Mary awakened late and rushed to the location. She ate her usual breakfast on the way to the race and felt great. She talked with Mark briefly before the start and ran behind him for the first mile. She was successful and completed the race a full twenty minutes after him only to find out that he had left. It was a wonderful feeling to finish the race so she began planning for her next event hoping to increase her speed and stamina by running three miles every day so she could finish with Mark at a race in the future.

1. Why did the author use the title "The Marathon" in the above passage?

    (A) to use as an instructional guide
    (B) as a repeating concept
    (C) to compare training methods
    (D) to review historical events

2. Which quote demonstrates the overall writing style demonstrated in the passage?

    (A) "trained by running six miles a day"
    (B) "only to find out that he had left"
    (C) "how great she was training"
    (D) "adequate hydration and carbohydrate loading"

3. Which message is most likely expressed in this passage?

   (A) Thoughtful preparation equals success.
   (B) Affection may increase your physical stamina.
   (C) There are gender differences between runners.
   (D) Training is the only way to succeed.

4. Which statement from the above passage expressed an opinion on training?

   (A) They stayed late to talk to her about how great she was training.
   (B) Her approach to training was different.
   (C) Adequate hydration and carbohydrate loading is needed.
   (D) She was successful and completed the race.

5. What is the topic sentence in the first paragraph?

   (A) She measured the exact distance from her home to run exactly three miles three days per week.
   (B) She signed up for the same five-kilometer race as Mark.
   (C) Mary was attracted to Mark.
   (D) It is common knowledge that all true athletes train in advance for competition.

6. Which of these statements is an example of Mary's failed logic regarding her athletic training?

   (A) she wanted to continue running
   (B) she will run three miles every day
   (C) she will stay up late before every race
   (D) running is a solitary sport

QUESTIONS 7 THROUGH 11 ARE BASED ON THE FOLLOWING PASSAGE.

Dietary Supplements and Health

A dietary supplement is a substance that is ingested to improve the overall health of the user. It would seem that a person with a healthy diet does not need supplements. Many people believe that these supplements make all the difference in their health. These supplements are costly products that require careful decision-making prior to consumption.

Vitamin supplements are stored by the body in varying concentrations. An excess of the supplement may result in adverse effects. In some of these supplements, the excess will be excreted resulting in a waste of money for the consumer. Many of these supplements contain ingredients that may be harmful if accumulated by the human body.

Consumers need to be aware of the supplements they are taking. Reputable internet sites should be searched for information on supplements and minimum daily requirements before purchase. Exaggerated claims of effects should be verified before purchasing a supplement. Some consumers will need supplements and should check with their health care provider before purchasing them. Most people will not need dietary supplements for health until the need is established. Consumer, beware and be smart!

7. What is the intent of the statement "Consumer, beware and be smart"?

    (A) to entertain the reader
    (B) to express feelings
    (C) to inform the reader
    (D) to persuade the reader

8. Which writing type would best reflect the title of the passage "Dietary Supplements and Health"?

    (A) expository
    (B) narrative
    (C) persuasive
    (D) technical

9. Which statement from the passage would identify this as a secondary source of information?

    (A) Exaggerated claims of effects should be verified before purchasing a supplement.
    (B) Most people will not need dietary supplements for health until the need is established.
    (C) Reputable internet sites should be searched for information on supplements and minimum daily requirements before purchase.
    (D) Consumer, beware and be smart!

10. "Vitamin supplements are stored by the body in varying concentrations." What is the text structure contained in this passage phrase?

    (A) sequence
    (B) cause and effect
    (C) comparison and contrast
    (D) description

11. "Consumers need to be aware of the supplements they are taking." Which choice best describes the term expressed in this quote?

    (A) topic
    (B) supporting detail
    (C) main idea
    (D) theme

My trip to England last year was unforgettable. From the beginning to the end it was as I expected. One particular characteristic of the people of the country made my trip memorable. The civility of the meeting participants was above reproach. Each time a question was asked the questioning participant would compliment the speaker, then expound on the inquiry and follow with a hearty "thank you so much." This approach to all presenters set the stage for all communication. This positive approach left me with a good feeling and an exemplar for my future interactions with others. The cost of travel and long hours on the plane was well offset by the lessons learned.

12. According to the above passage, what is the author's overall conclusion about this meeting?

    (A) Civility is a universal experience.
    (B) There are no advantages to international travel.
    (C) The time and work required to attend were not balanced by the benefits.
    (D) The traveler enjoyed this experience very much.

Tired of all the stress in the workplace? Why not offset the stress with bubble wrap popping. A new product has just been made available! Imagine the possibility of popping any time you wish. A great gift idea… the new bubble wrap key chain! Available now!

13. According to the above passage, what is the purpose of this advertisement?

    (A) to inform the buyer of a bargain
    (B) to persuade the buyer to purchase
    (C) to entertain the buyer to encourage purchase
    (D) to inform the reader about stress management

"As sold on TV" products are now available in many grocery and department stores. These items have been described as gadgets that are for a limited market and function. Even so, consumers are buying and enjoying the convenience of purchasing these items at their local retail store.

14. According to the above passage, what is the purpose of this article on the web?

    (A) to let the reader know of a new way to purchase the products
    (B) to persuade the reader to purchase the items online
    (C) to tell a great story about TV products
    (D) to excite the buyer

Charitable donations may be a great way to decrease income taxes next year. December seems to be the highest flow month for these contributions. This is probably due to the looming taxes to be paid. Maximizing charitable giving can help you by more than just creating a great feeling.

15. What is the tax information directed to the reader in the above passage?

    (A) Donations should be made to the government now.
    (B) December is the month to pay taxes.
    (C) Charitable donations can decrease income tax.
    (D) Donations increase your negative feelings about taxes.

Leadership is difficult in times of decrease. The challenges of success seem insurmountable. When the success of the company is in the upswing, leaders can fall into a more traditional role of compromising with other top leaders to sustain success. Maybe the goal should be fewer extreme swings in the trends rather than change toward the potential to loss or gain. For the leader, a moderate surplus along with moderate loss seems best.

16. What is the implied message regarding leadership in the above passage?

   (A) to praise the leader's accomplishments
   (B) to persuade the reader to avoid change
   (C) to give the reader insight into leadership
   (D) to exemplify leadership and moderation

The applicant for this open management role in the company brings a lifetime of experience to the role. He has been working in the field for fifteen years. His lifestyle and integrity match the needs of the company. Please consider his qualifications before considering other younger applicants.

17. What is the intended type of publication for the above passage?

   (A) company e-mail
   (B) newspaper
   (C) newsletter
   (D) internet advertisement

Obsessing on the Unattainable

James was an aspiring entrepreneur. He tired of people with negative feedback. His approach was different but consistent. "Why not?" was his mantra and call to action. Every investment opportunity was pursued, scrutinized, and decided upon. His approach to life was obsessively consistent.

A wealthy female investor asked him to invest in her. After many questions asked, private investigation, and scrutiny he agreed. Upon presenting the diamond ring to the investor and receiving a negative response he concluded that something needed to change in his life.

He decided upon a new perspective. "All of us would be better investors if we just made fewer decisions." (Daniel Kahneman)

18. What is meant by the quote at the end of the above passage?

   (A) Making decisions regarding money is dangerous.
   (B) Fewer decisions means more money.
   (C) Decisions make investing difficult.
   (D) Investments are better if made without excessive forethought.

This was a dual-center, randomized, wait-list controlled, prospective cohort pilot study involving forty baccalaureate students. All potential subjects were advised of standard options for dealing with stress other than this program.

19. Which type of literature is the above passage most likely from?

    (A) textbook
    (B) science fiction novel
    (C) research journal
    (D) mystery novel

QUESTIONS 20 AND 21 ARE BASED ON THE FOLLOWING E-MAIL WHICH WAS SENT TO A DIRECTOR OF HUMAN RESOURCES FROM A COMPANY EMPLOYEE.

Elizabeth,

I am writing to respond to the company policy regarding hiring into new positions that have not been posted within the system. I believe that management personnel are not being adequately informed and potential applicants are being ignored. We really want the best in our leadership team and ask that the policy be upheld at all costs.

20. What is the main purpose of the e-mail?

    (A) The author wants to question a policy.
    (B) The author wants to chat.
    (C) The author agrees with the current way that people are hired.
    (D) The author wants to be included in decisions involving the division.

21. What are the author's biases regarding the policy?

    (A) He is discussing the inadequacies of the division.
    (B) It is difficult to identify the author's bias.
    (C) He secretly believes that the policy is wrong.
    (D) There are no biases noted.

The nurse wants to provide care to the entire patient and not just parts. However some other medical professionals might concentrate on medicine based on aspects of the human condition. Two terms are commonly used to describe each approach. Disease is a total body problem and giving different medicines for different parts is not the best approach. Holistic medicine aspires to care for mind, body, and spirit, and holistic medicine attempts to care for the entire body.

22. What is the meaning of holistic in the passage above?

    (A) an approach with limitations or holes
    (B) caring for all aspects of the human condition
    (C) nursing care of aspects of the human condition
    (D) spiritual care

23. Read and follow the directions below.

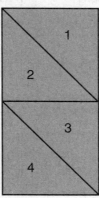

Step 1: Move triangle number 1 to the left of triangle number 2.
Step 2: Move triangle number 4 to the right of number 3.
Step 3: Rotate the figure 90 degrees.
What does the new shape look like?

(A)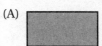

(B)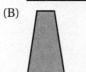

(C)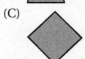

(D)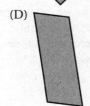

Hygiene	200
Key words	201
Rationale	209
Comfort	210
Key words	211
Rationale	219
Sleep	220
Key words	221
Rationale	230
Pain	231
Key words	232
Rationale	235

24. The reader is attempting to find information in a book by looking at the Table of Contents pictured above. On what page would the information about key words that relate to providing comfort be located?

(A) Page 201
(B) Page 209
(C) Page 211
(D) Page 220

From: Conference Committee

Sent: Wednesday, October 2, 2013 10:43 AM

Subject: Conference information

Dear Member,

The society invites you to join us February 12–15, 2014, in New Orleans, as we celebrate our 28th year of supporting and advancing integrative medicine at the 2014 Annual Conference. The Program Committee has planned a full program with scholarly papers, symposia, poster discussion sessions, posters, plenary sessions, and networking sessions.

We invite you to join us.

Registration is now open! Don't delay, register today!

---

25. According to the above email, how many events have been held by this organization?

(A) 7
(B) 14
(C) 15
(D) 28

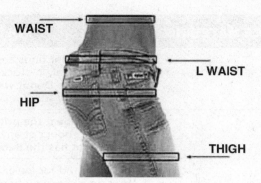

WAIST · L WAIST · HIP · THIGH

Size	Size	Hip																	Waist
24	0	Hip	32	33															23–24
25	1	Hip			34	35													24–25
26	3	Hip					36	37											25–26
27	5	Hip							38	39									26–27
28	7	Hip									40	41							27–28
29	9	Hip										41	42						28–29
30	11	Hip												43	44				29–30
31	13	Hip															45	46	30–32

SIZE CHART BY COUNTRY

New Dorinha Size	24	25	26	27	28	29	30	31
Dorinha Size	0	1	3	5	7	9	11	13
USA	00	0	2	4	6	8	10	12
USA (by Letter)	XXS	XS	XS	S	S	M	M	L
Brazil	34	36	38	40	42	44	46	48
Europe	28	30	32	34	36	38	40	42
UK	0	2	4	6	8	10	12	14
Japan	1	3	5	7	9	11	15	

26. The consumer is purchasing a new pair of pants online. According to the above sizing chart, which new size should be ordered if the hip measures 36 inches and the waist is 26 inches?

(A) 24

(B) 26

(C) 29

(D) 31

RETAILER	PRICE MATCHING?	POLICY
Home Depot	Yes	If the customer finds a current lower price on an identical, in-stock item from any retailer, Home Depot will match the price and beat it by 10%.
Lowe's	Yes	Lowe's will beat the price by 10% for an identical product at any local retail competitor that has the item in stock.
Office Depot	Yes	Must show ad for lower price at another store on a new, identical item. Office Depot will match the price at the time of purchase, or if the customer presents the ad within 14 days of the purchase, Office Depot will pay the difference.
OfficeMax	Yes	Must complete the OfficeMax online Price Match Request.
Sears	Yes	Sears will price match within 14 days of purchase, and beat the price by 10%.
Staples	Yes	Staples' price match guarantee applies to participating individual stores.
Target	Yes	Target will match prices within one week of purchase.
Wal-Mart	Yes	The store will offer price matching on an identical item before you make a purchase if you find an accurate lower price in an ad from a "local competitor." Internet pricing is excluded.

27. According to the above table, which retailers offer no guarantee in their price matching policy?

    (A) OfficeMax and Staples
    (B) Lowe's and Sears
    (C) Office Depot and Wal-Mart
    (D) Target and Home Depot

➢ **Toys—Retail**

AMERICAN FLYER TRAINS

    CENTRAL TELVSN & TRAINS

      4218 Calumt--------------------WE 2-2946

    DILDINE'S

      Factory Authorized Repair Service

      New & Used-Bought & Sold

      5711 Calumt--------------------WE 2-2495

BABYLAND HIRSCHBERG'S INC

    804 Bway Gary-----------------------Turnr 6-3685

CENTRAL TELVSN & TRAINS

    4218 Calumt Av--------------------WE 2-4964

DILDINE'S 5711 Calumt Av---------WE 2-2495

Gentry's Quality Hse

    All Toys-Sptg Gds-Applnces-Discounted

    5 Ridge Rd Munstr------------------TE 6-5066

    Goodyear Service Stores

    5706 Hohman Ave----------------WE 1-6625

McCAULEY'S VARIETY STORE

COMPLETE LINE OF TOYS – SUNDRIES –
SEWING SUPPLIES – AMERICAN GREETING
CARDS
Open Daily 9 AM to 9 PM
730 173rd--------------------------WE 2-1649

JACK & JILL SHOP

    Complete Year Round Selection

    6342 Ridge Rd Lansng----------GR 4-1100

JOE'S ELECTL SERVICE

    606 Burnhm Av CalCty---------TO 2-4470

  Lansing Hdw Co

    3263 Ridge Rd Lansng---------GR 4-2471

LIONEL TRAINS—

    CENTRAL TELVSN & TRAINS

      4218 Calumt Av--------------WE 2-4946

    DILDINE'S

      Factory Authorized Repair Service

      New & Used-Bought & Sold

      5711 Calumt------------------WE 2-2495

PEEWEE'S TOYS & HOBBIES

FREE TOY COUNSELING SERVICE

A Complete year-round Selection of Toys
Crafts & Hobby Supplies – Chemistry Sets
& Replacements – Pools – Wheel Goods

Trains – Hrs. 9:30 to 5:30
Mon. & Fri. 9:30 to 9:00

*Conveniently Located in the Heart of
the Highland Business District*

2835 Highway Ave Highland----TE 8-0663

---

28. What are the last four digits of the phone number for the free toy counseling service according to the Yellow Page ad?

(A) 1378

(B) 0663

(C) 5566

(D) 6917

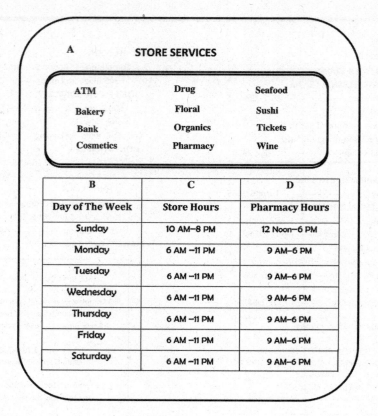

A	**STORE SERVICES**	
ATM	Drug	Seafood
Bakery	Floral	Sushi
Bank	Organics	Tickets
Cosmetics	Pharmacy	Wine

B	C	D
Day of The Week	Store Hours	Pharmacy Hours
Sunday	10 AM–8 PM	12 Noon–6 PM
Monday	6 AM –11 PM	9 AM–6 PM
Tuesday	6 AM –11 PM	9 AM–6 PM
Wednesday	6 AM –11 PM	9 AM–6 PM
Thursday	6 AM –11 PM	9 AM–6 PM
Friday	6 AM –11 PM	9 AM–6 PM
Saturday	6 AM –11 PM	9 AM–6 PM

29. Based on the above figure, in which section are store services posted?

(A) A
(B) B
(C) C
(D) D

Nutrition Facts

Serving Size 1 cup (228 g)
Servings Per Container 2

Amount Per Serving

Calories 250	Calories from Fat 110

	% **Daily Value***
Total Fat 12 g	19%
Saturated Fat 3 g	15%
Trans Fat 3 g	
Cholesterol 30 mg	10%
Sodium 470 mg	20%
Total Carbohydrate 31 g	10%
Dietary Fiber 0 g	0%
Sugars 5 g	
Protein 5 g	

Vitamin A	4%	●	Vitamin C	2%
Calcium	20%	●	Iron	4%

*Percent Daily Values are based on a 2,000 calorie diet. Your daily values may be higher or lower depending on your calorie needs.

30. A woman is keeping a diary of food and nutrient intake. She decided to consume a one-half serving of the food in the package. What should she enter on her diary?

(A) Calories   125
(B) Fiber   11 grams
(C) Sodium   21 milligrams
(D) Sugar   18 grams

We wanted to have a family reunion this year but found contacting all family members a challenge. We divided out the invitation list and wanted to send out the assignments to all locations. If you live in Massachusetts and your name begins with M–Z, please contact Lucy. All other residents of the state should contact Ken. If you live in New York State, contact Alisha if you live upstate. Mathew will be the contact person for New York City. We want to make sure all of you can participate in the activities planned and enjoy the fellowship. Please let us know if there are any issues with our usual Labor Day festivities, location, and time.

31. According to the above passage, who should Jack Anderson from Massachusetts contact for party information?

(A) Mathew
(B) Lucy
(C) Ken
(D) Alisha

Read the sentence and answer the question regarding the use of the underlined term.
In a rare moment of <u>lucidity</u>, the board of directors decided to rephrase the policy.

32. Which of the following is the best definition of the underlined word?

   (A) clarity
   (B) indecisiveness
   (C) lightheartedness
   (D) comprehensible

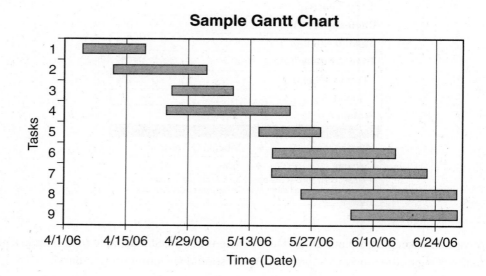

Sample Gantt Chart

33. The above graph was presented to the retention counselor to document time allocated for each assigned classroom task. Approximately how long will task #9 take?

   (A) 7 days
   (B) 15 days
   (C) 22 days
   (D) 30 days

Global Land—Ocean Temperature Index

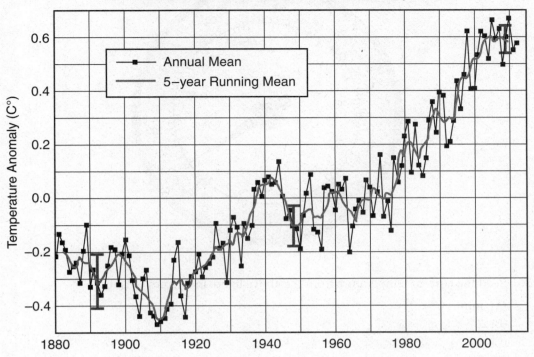

34. According to the above graph, how much have global temperatures increased since 1980?

    (A) −0.2
    (B) −0.4
    (C) 0.3
    (D) 0.5

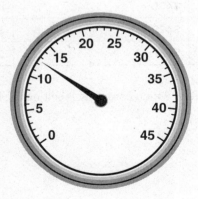

35. A measurement of approximately how many pounds is represented on the scale face above?

    (A) less than 1 pound
    (B) more than 5 pounds
    (C) more than 10 pounds
    (D) exactly 100 pounds

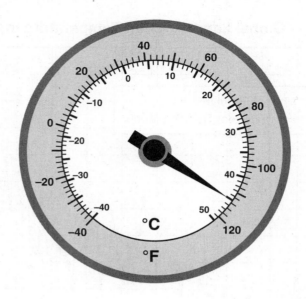

36. Read the current temperature from the above figure in degrees Celsius.

    (A) minus 5°
    (B) 20°
    (C) 45°
    (D) 70°

Online laptop computer cost comparison

STORE	PRICE	SHIPPING
HL	$405	$35
BB	$450	Included in price
A1	$425	$10
BRite	$415	$5

37. According to the above table, which company is selling the laptop computer at the lowest rate?

    (A) HL
    (B) BRite
    (C) BB
    (D) A1

QUESTIONS 38 AND 39 ARE BASED ON THE FOLLOWING TEXBOOK OUTLINE.

Section II Perspectives

Chapter 1 Overview

   Introduction

   Metastructure

   Future of science

Chapter 2 Standards

   Introduction

   What are standards

   Knowledge needs

   Specialty

   Future of standards

---

38. Identify a minor section of the outline.

   (A) Perspectives
   (B) Overview
   (C) Standards
   (D) Introduction

39. Identify a major section of the outline.

   (A) Perspectives
   (B) Metastructure
   (C) Future of science
   (D) What are standards

40. A student is interested in learning about becoming a dietitian. What would be the best location source to help him locate books on dietary therapy?

   (A) the national professional organization
   (B) online library catalog
   (C) a local hospital dietary department
   (D) his health care provider

QUESTIONS 41 AND 42 ARE BASED ON THE FOLLOWING PASSAGE.

David **requested**, I hope to have all of the family together this year in *Savannah, Georgia* for a reunion. He posted a memo in his blog site about that possibility.

41. In the above passage, what is the reason for the italics?

   (A) to denote the beginning of a dialogue
   (B) to draw attention to the place
   (C) to identify who is involved in the dialogue
   (D) to denote the ending of the story

42. What is the meaning of the bolding in the passage?

    (A) to denote a polite invitation
    (B) to draw attention to the passage
    (C) to identify an opinion
    (D) to denote the beginning of the memo

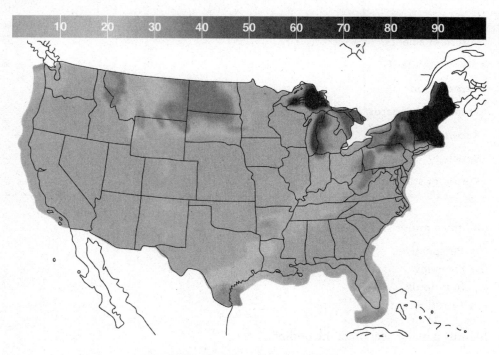

12 hour probable precipitation (%)

43. According to the above map, which regions of the United States are most likely to receive the heaviest rainfall or snow in the next twelve hours?

    (A) north central
    (B) south central
    (C) northwest
    (D) northeast

44. The guide words at the top of the page in a phone directory are "computers and contractors." What other business would be found on that page?

    (A) auto repair
    (B) concession supplies
    (C) coffee
    (D) compact disc

Sport club rates

	RACQUETBALL COURT 30 MINUTES WITH EQUIPMENT RENTAL	RACQUETBALL COURT 45 MINUTES WITH EQUIPMENT RENTAL	RACQUETBALL COURT 30 MINUTES WITHOUT EQUIPMENT
Mon–Fri	$25.00	$45.00	$15.00
Sat–Sun	$45.00	$60.00	$25.00
Early Bird Special	$15.00	$30.00	$12.00

45. Based on the above table, how much will it cost to play racquetball for thirty minutes on Wednesday evening? Your partner has the equipment.

    (A) $45.00
    (B) $30.00
    (C) $25.00
    (D) $15.00

Why work so hard to have ripped abdominal muscles? This new muscle contractor invention is easy and safe for men and women of ALL fitness levels to use. Just slip the belt around your waist, select your preferred mode, then advance through your day automatically developing your abs. You will feel the difference after each forty-minute workout.

46. What is the purpose of the above passage?

    (A) to persuade
    (B) to inform
    (C) to entertain
    (D) express feelings

ALASKA CRUISE	COST
1 A Wed–Thurs	$729.00
1 B Thurs–Fri	$769.00
2 A Fri–Sat	$769.00
2 B Tue–Wed	$729.00

47. There are two cruises leaving for Alaska in September. Amanda is determined to take the trip. Based on the above table, which trip should she choose if she has vacation Monday through Thursday that week and has $750 to spend?

    (A) 1 A
    (B) 1 B
    (C) 2 A
    (D) 2 B

Chapter 3: Flowers of Europe

1. Variations

2. Where to locate them

    a. England

    b. Ireland

    c. Australia

    d. Spain

    e. France

48. Based on the pattern of the outline above, what is the most confusing entry?

    (A) England
    (B) Australia
    (C) Ireland
    (D) France

Part 2: Mathematics

Time: 51 minutes

34 questions

1. Simplify the expression: $(3+(4\times[5-2]))$

   (A) 21
   (B) 33
   (C) 15
   (D) 9

2. Simplify the expression: $(3+2)^2-7$

   (A) 19
   (B) 18
   (C) 12
   (D) 9

3. Simplify the expression: $532-79$

   (A) 453
   (B) 42
   (C) 316
   (D) 441

4. Simplify the expression: $1050-105$

   (A) 105
   (B) 905
   (C) 945
   (D) 0

5. A student nurse must give a patient 225 milligrams (mg) of a drug. The drug is supplied in 75 mg tablets. How many tablets should the patient receive?

   (A) 2 tablets
   (B) 3 tablets
   (C) $2\frac{1}{2}$ tablets
   (D) $1\frac{1}{2}$ tablets

6. A man wants to replace the damaged fence bordering his house to keep his dogs from getting out. The boundary is a line that measures 6 feet wide by 250 feet long. Fencing costs $20 per foot. How much will the fence cost to replace?

(A) $16,800
(B) $12,800
(C) $5,120
(D) $1,560

7. What is the sum of $\frac{3}{6} + \frac{2}{3}$?

(A) $\frac{5}{12}$

(B) $\frac{9}{18}$

(C) $\frac{5}{9}$

(D) $\frac{7}{6}$

8. What is the product of $4\frac{1}{3} \times \frac{6}{3}$?

(A) $\frac{3}{9}$

(B) $8\frac{2}{3}$

(C) $\frac{39}{9}$

(D) $\frac{18}{8}$

9. Simplify the expression: 0.422×6.13

(A) 25.87
(B) 1.264
(C) 2.587
(D) 0.026

10. Which of the following decimals is an approximate equivalent to $\sqrt{7}$?

(A) 2.64
(B) 2.70
(C) 2.55
(D) 2.44

11. What percent of 100 is 0.007?

(A) 7%
(B) 0.7%
(C) 0.07%
(D) 70%

12. Which of the following decimals is equivalent to the expression $\frac{45}{625}$?

    (A) 13.89

    (B) 1.389

    (C) 0.072

    (D) 0.086

13. Which of the following numbers is the largest?

    (A) $\frac{4}{7}$

    (B) $\frac{5}{6}$

    (C) $\frac{19}{30}$

    (D) $\frac{45}{60}$

14. Estimate the product of $8{,}765 \times 47$.

    (A) 399,399

    (B) 450,500

    (C) 400,500

    (D) 411,955

15. Reconcile this checking account for this month. The previous balance was $6,544.25. Deposits were made for $3,500.50 and $240.75. Checks were written for $1,475 and $2,250. What is the remaining balance?

    (A) $10,285.50

    (B) $7,470.75

    (C) $6,560.50

    (D) $8,574.75

16. An employee earns $29.21 per hour, works three 12-hour shifts per week, and is paid every two weeks. Deductions each pay period include: $565.13 taxes, $100.22 retirement plan, and $125.15 health insurance. What is this employee's take-home pay every two weeks?

    (A) $1,421.26

    (B) $1,312.62

    (C) $1,262.42

    (D) $1,351.66

17. A visitor has lunch at a hospital cafeteria and decides on the day's special including a bowl of soup and garlic bread for $3.25. If the visitor adds two medium drinks for $1.25 each and a slice of pie for $1.50, how much will the total lunch cost?

    (A) $7.25

    (B) $5.45

    (C) $6.75

    (D) $6.00

18. A local catered luncheon is planned for which 150 reservations have been received, including 125 over age twelve and 25 under age twelve. The luncheon cost for those under twelve is $15 and for those above twelve, $30. Which of the following is the cost of the luncheon?

(A) $4,500
(B) $4,125
(C) $3,125
(D) $262

19. An artisan is making an item consisting of $\frac{1}{5}$ plastic, $\frac{1}{75}$ metal, $\frac{1}{15}$ nylon, and the rest is textile material. What fraction of the item consists of textile material?

(A) $\frac{66}{150}$

(B) $\frac{45}{150}$

(C) $\frac{25}{90}$

(D) $\frac{54}{75}$

20. The 12 students who received an A in their first biology exam made up 9% of the students in the class. Find the total number of students in the class.

(A) 128
(B) 133
(C) 121
(D) 108

21. A club has 15 male and 106 female members. What is the ratio of male to female members in the club?

(A) 12:88
(B) 25:75
(C) 10:90
(D) 30:70

22. This masterpiece has its first printing date written as 1611. What is this date in Roman numerals?

(A) MDX
(B) MDXII
(C) MDCXI
(D) MDIX

23. A museum displayed an ancient silver coin dated MCXCVIII. What is this date in conventional numbers?

(A) 1918
(B) 1198
(C) 1247
(D) 1194

24. The volunteers were told that the charity walk consisted of 12 kilometers. How many miles would that be?

(A) 12.5
(B) 9.54
(C) 19.2
(D) 7.44

25. The dieter was told to drink 270 milliliters of water per day. How much would that be in fluid ounces?

(A) 21
(B) 9
(C) 15
(D) 24

26. A metalworker has a 5-ft pipe from which he must cut two smaller pieces: one 30 inches long and the other 14 inches long. What would be the appropriate measuring tool to use?

(A) caliper
(B) ruler
(C) yardstick
(D) beaker

27. A scale model map assigns 15,000 miles to 1 inch. If the distance from earth to moon measures 16 inches on the map, how far is this distance?

(A) 240,000
(B) 250,000
(C) 300,500
(D) 360,000

28. In the theory, "Quality of sleep impacts a worker's job performance," what is the dependent variable?

(A) job
(B) performance
(C) quality
(D) sleep

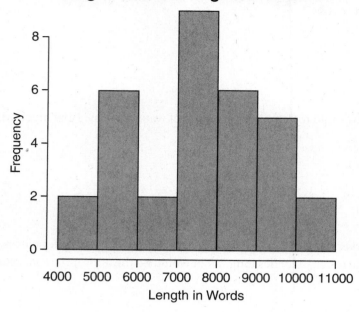

Length of Greek Tragedies in Words

29. Based on the above graph above, which range represents the most frequent length in words of Greek tragedies?
    (A) 4,000–11,000
    (B) 5,000–6,000
    (C) 7,000–8,000
    (D) 8,000–9,000

GRADE	NUMBER OF STUDENTS
A	13
B	57
C	34
D	9
E	3

30. The grade distribution on an examination for a class of students is shown in the above table. If the data were transcribed into a pie chart, what fraction of the circle would represent the number of students who received an A on the exam?

    (A) $\dfrac{1}{2}$

    (B) $\dfrac{1}{3}$

    (C) $\dfrac{1}{8}$

    (D) $\dfrac{1}{11}$

31. Simplify the expression: $(2x+3)(4x-5)$

   (A) $8x^2+2x-15$
   (B) $-8x^2+12x$
   (C) $8x^2+22x+5$
   (D) $10x^2-8x+8$

32. Express the following phrase into a mathematical expression: Marla is five years older than her sister; if Marla's age is m, what is the sum of their ages?

   (A) $m+5=x$
   (B) $2m+5=x$
   (C) $2m-5=x$
   (D) $5m-5=x$

33. Solve this equation for z: $5(3z+2)=6z-8$

   (A) 2
   (B) −2
   (C) −3
   (D) 4

34. Solve the inequality: $|x-20|>15$

   (A) $x<1$ and $x>6$
   (B) $x<5$ and $x>10$
   (C) $x<-5$ or $x>5$
   (D) $x<5$ or $x>35$

Part 3: Science

Time: 66 minutes

54 questions

QUESTIONS 1 AND 2 ARE BASED ON THE PERIODIC TABLE.

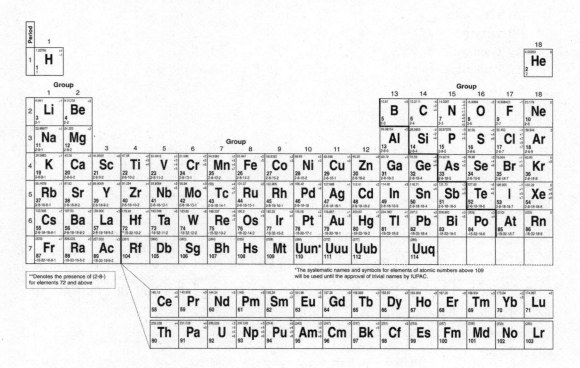

1. Which element would have the highest atomic mass?

   (A) In
   (B) Sn
   (C) N
   (D) O

2. How many protons would a positively charged isotope ion of O-18 have?

   (A) 8
   (B) 9
   (C) 10
   (D) 12

3. One morning two observers are looking toward the rising sun. One of these observers is in Brazil; the other, in Canada. In which direction must they look to see the rising sun?

(A) The observer in Brazil must look westward while the other must look eastward.
(B) Both observers must look eastward.
(C) The observer in Canada must look westward while the other must look eastward.
(D) Both observers must look westward.

4. Which statement best describes kinetic energy?

(A) energy based on mass
(B) energy based on motion
(C) energy based on chemical properties
(D) stored energy

5. What is a protein catalyst that lowers energy activation in living organisms?

(A) substrate
(B) enzyme
(C) coenzyme
(D) catalyst

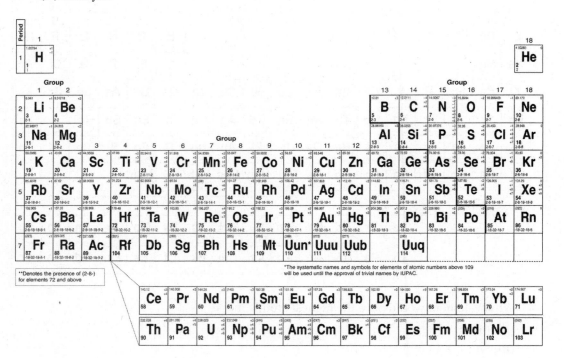

6. Referring to the above periodic table, complete this sentence.

If you have an element that has 20 protons, 21 neutrons, and 18 electrons, this atom would have a charge of _____ and an atomic weight of_____.

(A) +2, 41
(B) −2, 38
(C) +2, 38
(D) −2, 41

7. The alkali metals are located in the far left column of the periodic chart. What is their primary chemical affinity?

(A) They have two electrons in their outer orbit.
(B) They become less active as you progress from the top elements to the bottom.
(C) They want to take up electrons from other binding elements.
(D) They are very active with a single electron in their outer orbit.

8. A solution has a hydrogen ion activity of 1 part per 10,000. What is the pH of the solution?

(A) pH 12.5
(B) pH 1
(C) pH 7
(D) pH 4

9. What is the difference between saturated and unsaturated hydrocarbons?

(A) The saturated ones have double bonds.
(B) The saturated ones are called alkenes.
(C) The unsaturated ones are called alkynes.
(D) The unsaturated ones allow attachments to unbounded carbon.

10. Which of these Lewis structure diagrams would be the closest representation of sulfur dioxide?

(A) $\ddot{O}=\ddot{S}=\ddot{O}$

(B) $:\ddot{O}-\ddot{S}=\ddot{O}$

(C) $:\ddot{O}-\ddot{S}=\ddot{O}$

(D) $:\ddot{O}-\ddot{S}=\ddot{O}:$

11. Choose the answer that shows the balanced equation for:
    ___FeS+___$O_2 \rightarrow$ ___Fe_2O_3 +___SO_2

(A) $3\ FeS + 2\ O_2 \rightarrow 3\ Fe_2O_3 + 2\ SO_2$
(B) $4\ FeS + 7\ O_2 \rightarrow 2\ Fe_2O_3 + 4\ SO_2$
(C) $3\ FeS + O_2 \rightarrow 6\ Fe_2O_3 + 2\ SO_2$
(D) $FeS + O_2 \rightarrow 2\ Fe_2O_3 + SO_2$

12. What is the pH of water?

(A) 2
(B) 6
(C) 7
(D) 9

13. What needs to be present when solids convert to a liquid state?

(A) change in temperature
(B) atomic motion
(C) change in environment
(D) a crystalline structure

14. Which of these is the most important reason to do scientific research?

   (A) helps to improve the human condition
   (B) to discover truth
   (C) advancement of human knowledge
   (D) to use the information for new applications of science

15. Identify the purpose of this sentence: "Students want to get advanced degrees once they start in an educational program."

   (A) directional hypothesis
   (B) non-directional hypothesis
   (C) a scientific argument
   (D) a research interest

16. This research study is in progress. At what step of the scientific process is this research team? A team is investigating the effects of garlic on stored beef. They have stated the hypothesis as: "garlic extract is effective as a natural food preservative." They have begun injecting beef with the extract and monitoring the refrigerator shelf life of the beef.

   (A) hypothesis development
   (B) data collection
   (C) analysis
   (D) conclusion

17. Which research variable is the presumed effect?

   (A) independent
   (B) dependent
   (C) both independent and dependent
   (D) neither independent nor dependent

18. In a study called "What is the effect of radon on health?" what is the independent variable?

   (A) radon
   (B) health
   (C) effect
   (D) both radon and health

19. A group of elderly people were questioned about their experience in a long term care facility. The study was stopped when the researchers felt they were getting the same responses or the data collection was saturated. What type of research design is this?

   (A) either qualitative or quantitative
   (B) quantitative
   (C) qualitative
   (D) mixed design

20. A researcher is exploring the thought that there may be an issue contributing to a phenomenon that has never been explored before. What type of reasoning is this?

    (A) quantitative
    (B) extraneous
    (C) inductive
    (D) proactive

21. The research team is considering a double blind study. Which of these designs would fit?

    (A) non-experimental design
    (B) qualitative design
    (C) experimental design
    (D) survey

22. The researchers are attempting to test a scientific model. What would give the highest confidence in a theoretical model?

    (A) The research has been repeated many times with different subjects with the same results.
    (B) The model fails the test in one area of the intervention.
    (C) There is a researcher bias.
    (D) The instrument is accurate and reflects the model's assumptions.

23. This research was repeated many times but there are major differences in the data collected across samples. What is the problem with the design?

    (A) the independent variable
    (B) the dependent variable
    (C) an extraneous variable
    (D) the confounding variable

24. Where is a cell's genetic information contained?

    (A) ribosome
    (B) mitochondria
    (C) nucleolus
    (D) nucleus

25. A couple has two children, one child with an autosomal dominant disease trait and one normal child. The father is affected by the disease but the mother is not. What is the possibility that the next child will be affected?

    (A) 50%
    (B) 33%
    (C) 25%
    (D) cannot be predicted

26. Which of these biological classifications are listed in correct hierarchical order?

   (A) domain, kingdom, species, genus
   (B) phyllum, class, order, family
   (C) genus, species, family, order
   (D) domain, kingdom, family, class

27. What gene structure determines the mutations in DNA?

   (A) RNA
   (B) alleles
   (C) nitrogenous base
   (D) nucleic acid

28. What are the names of the proteins in nitrogenous bases in DNA?

   (A) adenine, cytosine, guanine, thymine
   (B) pentose, purine, phosphate, ribose
   (C) pyrimidine, uracil, purine, guanine
   (D) uracil, adenine, guanine, cystocine

29. What is the function of cellular mitochondria?

   (A) allow substances in and out of cells
   (B) organize and segregate the chromosomes
   (C) location for production of ATP
   (D) transport of protein

30. What is the primary differentiating structure of plant cells that are different from animal cells?

   (A) large vacuoles
   (B) no mitochondria
   (C) soft cell wall
   (D) ribosomes

31. What is the output of meiosis?

   (A) two cells
   (B) six cells
   (C) pairs of sister chromatids
   (D) genetic variability

32. Several chemotherapy agents stop cancer growth by altering the reproductive process and slowing the rapid reproduction of cells. How does chemotherapy most likely work?

   (A) enzymes would not be blocked
   (B) RNA function could be enhanced
   (C) protein formulation could be increased
   (D) the phases in cell replication could be halted

33. Where is the DNA located in prokaryotic cells?

    (A) nucleolus
    (B) cell wall
    (C) ribosomes
    (D) nucleoid

34. What substance is required to translate DNA codes into protein?

    (A) ribosome
    (B) ribonucleic acid
    (C) chromosomes
    (D) genes

35. What is a risk factor for Down's Syndrome Trisomy 21?

    (A) increased paternal age
    (B) mutagens in the uterus
    (C) family history
    (D) pregnancy in women over age 35

36. When is active acquired immunity gained?

    (A) in the pregnant uterus
    (B) after birth
    (C) with immunizations
    (D) in adult years

37. Of the four tissue types in the human body, which one does not have its own blood supply?

    (A) epithelial
    (B) connective
    (C) muscular
    (D) nervous

38. Which system works with the respiratory system to regulate respiratory rate and depth?

    (A) muscular system
    (B) nervous system
    (C) skeletal system
    (D) endocrine system

39. How do neurotransmitters interact with the postsynaptic membrane?

    (A) by binding to a receptor
    (B) by binding to a Nissl body
    (C) by binding to a glial cell
    (D) by binding to a neurofibril

40. A person has been diagnosed with a brain tumor. Where would the tumor be located if the client is having alterations in heart rate and blood pressure?

(A) medulla oblongata
(B) pons
(C) midbrain
(D) cerebrum

41. A group of mountain climbers have experienced confusion, tachycardia, edema, and decreased renal output after climbing a mountain in the West. Why would they develop these problems?

(A) bronchoconstriction
(B) hypoventilation
(C) decreased inspired oxygen
(D) diffusion abnormalities

42. A man with a thirty-year history of smoking was diagnosed with lung cancer. He was exposed to air pollution, asbestos, and radiation at his job. What was probably the cause of his cancer?

(A) air pollution
(B) asbestos
(C) cigarette smoke
(D) radiation

43. A thirty-two-year-old female suffers from severe brain damage following a motor vehicle accident. After returning home she notices that her thought processes and goal-oriented behavior are impaired. What area of the brain was probably injured?

(A) thalamus
(B) limbic
(C) prefrontal
(D) occipital

44. Which chamber of the heart has the highest pressure?

(A) right atrium
(B) left atrium
(C) left ventricle
(D) right ventricle

45. What structure does oxygenated blood flow through?

(A) superior vena cava
(B) pulmonary veins
(C) pulmonary artery
(D) cardiac veins

46. What is the difference between cardiac and skeletal muscle?

(A) Cardiac muscle cells are arranged in branching networks.
(B) Skeletal muscle cells have only one nucleus.
(C) Cardiac muscle cells appear striped.
(D) Skeletal muscle cells contain sarcomeres.

47. Which hormone promotes breast development during puberty?

(A) progesterone
(B) prolactin
(C) oxytocin
(D) estrogen

48. Which of these functions belong to the renal system?

(A) absorption of digested food
(B) chemical breakdown of food particles
(C) micturition
(D) mechanical breakdown of food particles

49. What immunoglobulin is in the saliva?

(A) IgG
(B) IgD
(C) IgE
(D) IgA

50. What does parasympathetic stimulation to the pancreas accomplish?

(A) hormonal inhibition
(B) enzyme secretion
(C) vasoconstriction
(D) decreased bicarbonate production

51. What is free bilirubin converted to in the liver?

(A) unconjugated bilirubin
(B) biliverdin
(C) conjugated bilirubin
(D) urobilinogen

52. What would cause an allergic reaction to occur in a person who has a penicillin allergy?

(A) beta-adrenergic agonists
(B) histamine
(C) calcium
(D) cortisol

53. Which burn is the most painful?

    (A) first degree
    (B) superficial partial-thickness
    (C) deep partial-thickness
    (D) third degree

54. What is the scientific name of male pattern baldness?

    (A) alopecia
    (B) areata
    (C) hirsutism
    (D) paronychia

Part 4: English and Language Usage

Time: 34 minutes

34 questions

1. John _____ kind words to Joan.

   Which of the following options correctly completes the sentence above?

   (A) his
   (B) spoke
   (C) speak
   (D) has

2. Jake, upon receiving the startling news, suddenly cancelled the trip.

   Which of the following correctly identifies the parts of speech in the underlined portions of the sentence above?

   (A) subject; clause
   (B) noun; pronoun
   (C) noun; object
   (D) pronoun; adverb

3. Which of the following sentences has correct subject–verb agreement?

   (A) When arriving to the restaurant, she finding the restroom first.
   (B) The reunion often lingers, the family then retreat for the day.
   (C) The club seems merit-based until everyone gets awards for just showing up.
   (D) When I wants silence, the neighbors give me mayhem.

4. Which of the following sentences provides an example of correct subject–verb agreement?

   (A) The faculty, upon analyzing applicant records, accept only the top 100.
   (B) The team of participants are performing in orchestrated harmony.
   (C) The group of cyclist, viewing the intricate map, choose the alternate trail.
   (D) The crowd, pleased with the show, cheers until the band comes back.

5. When Sally consented for Sam to visit, ___ hoped he would take a shortcut.

   Which of the following options is the correct pronoun for the sentence above? The antecedent of the pronoun to be added is underlined.

   (A) him
   (B) she
   (C) he
   (D) her

6. While strolling with lissome Dally and Dilly, Dan was stopped often by neighbors desiring to pet ___ dogs.

Which of the following is the correct pronoun to complete the sentence above?

(A) it
(B) he's
(C) his
(D) its

7. Which of the following is an example of correctly punctuated direct dialogue sentence?

(A) Lois told me, "she might go out with me sometime again soon."
(B) She told me that "she might go out with me sometime again soon."
(C) Lois told me, "Maybe we can go out sometime again soon."
(D) She told me, maybe we can go out sometime again soon.

8. Which of the following sentences correctly punctuates direct dialogue?

(A) "Over any other 'literary style,' I prefer to 'read fiction,'" confided Sandy.
(B) I prefer to "read fiction, confided" Sandy, over "any other" literary style.
(C) Sally confided, "I prefer to read fiction over any other literary style."
(D) Sally confided that she preferred to read fiction over any other literary style.

9. Which of the following is an example of second-person point of view?

(A) The couple decided to leave the concert as soon as the last song started to avoid the heavy traffic.
(B) We thought it better to leave the concert toward the start of the last song to avoid the heavy traffic.
(C) I and my date decided to leave the concert when the last song started to avoid the heavy traffic.
(D) You have to decide to leave the concert at the start of the last song to avoid the heavy traffic.

10. Which of the following sentences in the instructions below is an example of first-person voice?

(A) Once anyone sees the curve, it is easy to make the right and quick left turns.
(B) After we saw the curve, we failed to see the way to turn right and then left.
(C) As soon as you see the curve, make a right and then a quick left turn.
(D) As soon as he missed the curve, there was no way to turn right and then left.

11. Kane and Kate worked on a fence project. The supplies ran out. He checked the storeroom. She contacted the neighbors.

Which of the following options best uses grammar for style and clarity to combine the sentences above?

(A) Kane and Kate worked on a fence project when the supplies ran out; he checked the storeroom, and she contacted the neighbors.

(B) While Kane and Kate worked on a fence project, the supplies ran out; he checked the storeroom while she contacted the neighbors.

(C) The supplies ran out while Kane and Kate worked on a fence project; he checked the storeroom, but she contacted the neighbors.

(D) The supplies ran out while they worked on a fence project; Kate contacted the neighbors while Kane checked the storeroom.

12. We landed at the mountainside. The skies were clear. The wind was glacial. We did not hike.

Which of the following options best uses grammar for style and clarity to combine the sentences above?

(A) The skies were clear when we landed at the mountainside, but we did not hike because the wind was glacial.

(B) We landed at the mountainside, the skies were clear and the wind was glacial, so we did not hike.

(C) When we landed at the mountainside, the skies were clear; however, since the wind was glacial, we did not hike.

(D) When we landed at the mountainside, the skies were clear; since the wind was glacial, we did not hike.

13. In line with his wayfarer friends, he was a vagabond.

Which of the following is the meaning of the word *vagabond* as used in the sentence above?

(A) borrower and debtor

(B) bondholder and creditor

(C) vagrant and wanderer

(D) resident and dweller

14. After his adversity was over, he decided to be more circumspect.

Which of the following is the meaning of the word *circumspect*?

(A) pleasant

(B) cautious

(C) outspoken

(D) well-rounded

15. The patient's condition showed all the sultry symptoms of hyperthermia.

    In the sentence above, the prefix *hyper-* indicates that the condition was related to what type of problem?

    (A) overexcited behavior
    (B) nervous appearance
    (C) high temperature
    (D) low blood pressure

16. The students pondered into the morning hours about the latest lecture on pathophysiology.

    In the sentence above, the suffix *–ology* can best be defined by which of the following words?

    (A) state or condition
    (B) belief in
    (C) a part of
    (D) study of

17. Which of the following words is spelled correctly?

    (A) concieve
    (B) benefitial
    (C) accompanied
    (D) disipate

18. Which of the following words is spelled correctly?

    (A) ridiculos
    (B) symmetry
    (C) tiranny
    (D) unanymous

19. She was closer to paying off the _____, with the interest bulk paid, and she no longer worried about debt.

    Which of the following options correctly completes the sentence above?

    (A) principle
    (B) principal
    (C) capital
    (D) capitol

20. I found _____ belongings if _____ interested.

    Which of the following options correctly completes the question above?

    (A) you're; you
    (B) your; you's
    (C) your; you're
    (D) you're; your

21. Paul said to them, <u>accept</u> these abide in the ship, you cannot be saved.

    Which of the following words corrects the spelling of the underlined word in the sentence above?

    (A) exert
    (B) eccept
    (C) exempt
    (D) except

22. Which of the following underlined words is an example of correct spelling?

    (A) Because her hair took longer in <u>dyeing</u>, her beautician kept her longer.
    (B) Her unconventional <u>genera</u> of novel writing was puzzling.
    (C) Because of the <u>stationery</u> nature of the road, he arrived late to the meeting.
    (D) Despite your usual tardiness, <u>your</u> here early today.

23. Which of the following sentences follows the rules of capitalization?

    (A) I like the month of june.
    (B) I am with uncle Pete.
    (C) I am from the Old South.
    (D) I'll be back in Spring.

24. When we visit South America, we'd like to admire Machu Picchu, the ancient ruins of the Incas, and a mysterious waterside, such as lake Titicaca.

    Which of the following words in the sentence above should be capitalized?

    (A) ruins
    (B) mysterious
    (C) waterside
    (D) lake

25. Which of the following sentences correctly applies the rules of punctuation?

    (A) We promised to arrive on time, therefore; we set the alarm clock to ring before sunrise.
    (B) We promised to arrive on time; therefore, we set the alarm clock to ring before sunrise.
    (C) We promised to arrive on time, therefore, we set the alarm clock to ring before sunrise.
    (D) We promised to arrive on time; therefore we set the alarm clock to ring before sunrise.

26. I finished the project last night between computer anomalies __ while this has happened before, this time they were worse.

    Which of the following punctuation marks correctly completes the sentence above?

    (A) …
    (B) ,
    (C) ;
    (D) :

27. Which of the following is an example of a simple sentence?

(A) The student who waited long.
(B) Missed the deadline.
(C) The student who was late, waited long, and missed the deadline.
(D) The student waited long, was late, and missed the deadline.

28. Which of the following is an example of a simple sentence?

(A) The parrot of the beautiful blue stripes had squawked for a long while, although I gave him a fresh bunch of red grapes.
(B) The parrot of the beautiful blue stripes had squawked for a long while, but he started talking when I gave him a fresh bunch of red grapes.
(C) The parrot of the beautiful blue stripes had squawked for a long while until I gave him a fresh bunch of red grapes.
(D) The parrot of the beautiful blue stripes had squawked for a long while but started talking with a fresh bunch of red grapes.

29. The tourist gazed through the shopping mall. She was amazed at the countless bargains on display.

Which of the following uses a conjunction to combine the sentences above so that the focus is more on the tourist's gazing through the mall and less on her amazement?

(A) The tourist gazed through the shopping mall, since she was amazed at the countless bargains on display.
(B) The tourist gazed through the shopping mall and was amazed at the countless bargains on display.
(C) As the tourist gazed through the shopping mall, she was amazed at the countless bargains on display.
(D) The tourist gazed through the shopping mall; she was amazed at the countless bargains on display.

30. The student who makes the highest grades _____

Which of the following completes the above into a simple sentence?

(A) reads all assignments, and some find her friendly.
(B) reads all assignments and occasionally socializes.
(C) reads all assignments, although finds no time for socializing.
(D) reads all assignments after her close friends socialize with her.

31. Which of the following sentences is most clear and correct?

(A) When the timer was just about to toll the last student turned in the test.
(B) The last student turned in the test when the timer was just about to toll.
(C) The last student turned in the test near timer toll.
(D) About timer-toll the last student turned in the test.

32. We planned to visit mom. The rain came down. The weatherman said it would last a week. We cancelled the trip.

    To improve sentence fluency, which of the following best states the information above in a single sentence?

    (A) As we planned to visit mom, the rain came down and the weatherman said it would last a week, so we cancelled the trip.
    (B) As we planned to visit mom and the rain came down, the weatherman said it would last a week, so we cancelled the trip.
    (C) When the rain came down and the weatherman said it would last a week, we cancelled the trip we planned to visit mom.
    (D) We planned to visit mom but the rain came down, when the weatherman said it would last a week we cancelled the trip.

33. I went sightseeing. I could not turn back. I spent the daylight hours driving. I got lost.

    To improve sentence fluency, which of the following best states the information above in a single sentence?

    (A) I went sightseeing and I could not turn back, so I spent the daylight hours driving and got lost.
    (B) I went sightseeing, but I could not turn back, so I spent the daylight hours driving, and I got lost.
    (C) I got lost because I spent the daylight hours driving, since I could not turn back when I went sightseeing.
    (D) I spent the daylight hours driving and I got lost because I went sightseeing, and I could not turn back.

34. We went camping. The children joined us. We lost track of time. We stayed over.

    To improve sentence fluency, which of the following best states the information above in a single sentence?

    (A) We went camping, and the children joined us, we lost track of time, so we stayed over.
    (B) We went camping and the children joined us, we stayed over because we lost track of time.
    (C) When we went camping the children joined us, and we lost track of time as we stayed over.
    (D) The children joined us when we went camping and, because we lost track of time, we stayed over.

ANSWER KEY
Practice Test 2

READING

1. B	13. B	25. D	37. B
2. B	14. A	26. B	38. D
3. A	15. C	27. A	39. A
4. C	16. D	28. B	40. B
5. D	17. A	29. A	41. B
6. B	18. D	30. A	42. A
7. D	19. C	31. C	43. D
8. C	20. A	32. A	44. B
9. B	21. A	33. C	45. D
10. D	22. B	34. D	46. A
11. B	23. D	35. C	47. D
12. D	24. C	36. C	48. B

MATHEMATICS

1. C	10. A	19. D	28. B
2. B	11. B	20. B	29. C
3. A	12. C	21. A	30. C
4. C	13. B	22. C	31. A
5. B	14. D	23. B	32. C
6. C	15. C	24. D	33. B
7. D	16. B	25. B	34. D
8. B	17. A	26. C	
9. C	18. B	27. A	

SCIENCE

1. B	15. D	29. C	43. C
2. A	16. B	30. A	44. C
3. B	17. B	31. D	45. B
4. B	18. A	32. D	46. A
5. B	19. C	33. D	47. D
6. A	20. C	34. B	48. C
7. D	21. C	35. D	49. D
8. D	22. A	36. C	50. B
9. D	23. C	37. A	51. C
10. B	24. D	38. B	52. B
11. B	25. A	39. A	53. B
12. C	26. B	40. A	54. A
13. B	27. B	41. C	
14. D	28. A	42. C	

ENGLISH AND LANGUAGE USAGE

1. B	10. B	19. B	28. D
2. C	11. C	20. C	29. A
3. C	12. A	21. D	30. B
4. D	13. C	22. A	31. B
5. B	14. B	23. C	32. C
6. C	15. C	24. D	33. C
7. C	16. D	25. B	34. D
8. C	17. C	26. C	
9. D	18. B	27. C	

ANSWER EXPLANATIONS
Reading

1. **(B)** The title represents the theme of the passage as a repeating concept. The topic and main idea was the comparison of training for an athletic event. The detail unfolded during the entire passage.

2. **(B)** The quote represents a narrative style of telling a story. The passage was a narrative; the other answers demonstrate how details are presented to support the story.

3. **(A)** This is the general idea expressed by the author. The other choices reflect more specific behaviors and supporting details.

4. **(C)** The author suggests that adequate hydration and carbohydrate loading is needed for training. The passage compares two different types of training for an athletic event. The other responses represent some aspects of training but are not expressed as opinions.

5. **(D)** The topic sentence is usually the first sentence and expresses the main point of the paragraph or passage. The paragraph was comparing two types of training for a marathon. The other responses were supporting details for the story.

6. **(B)** Mary believes that running three miles every day is the best way to train for a marathon. The author does not mention the other conclusions.

7. **(D)** This passage was intended to persuade the reader about the use of dietary supplements. Poetry is often used to evoke emotions. Fiction entertains the reader. The author was not trying to describe a particular practice of health care.

8. **(C)** Persuasive writing tries to convince the reader to agree with the author. Expository passages explain a topic or subject in order to increase understanding of ideas. Technical writing usually addresses precise information. Narrative style tells a story.

9. **(B)** The answer is most likely from a primary source. Therefore the stem of the question is a secondary statement type.

10. **(D)** The passage describes the use of dietary supplements in health care. A sequence is usually expressed as a bulleted or numbered list. A comparison–contrast structure has two opposing ideas that force the reader to identify a difference. A cause and effect structure would describe an event with expected consequences.

11. **(B)** This is a supporting detail expressed by the author. The statement is too specific to be an overall topic, main idea, or theme.

12. **(D)** The overall intent of the passage is to express the author's opinion on balance of benefit to expense on attending a meeting. The other answers do not mention an overall experience; instead they focus on specific experiences, or express emotions and feelings opposite to the statements in the passage.

13. **(B)** The passage is an advertisement and is selling a product. This passage was meant to persuade the reader to make the purchase.

14. **(A)** The passage seems to be from the business section of a newspaper. The author was not trying to persuade you to purchase something or trying to get you to laugh. Most business articles provide straightforward information.

15. **(C)** This article summarizes the impact of charitable donations and income tax. All other answers are counter to the perspective of the author.

16. **(D)** The overall purpose is for the reader to compare–contrast leadership and moderation.

17. **(A)** This is a justification for hiring a particular candidate for a company role and would be sent via e-mail.

18. **(D)** The quote draws attention to the relationship between investments and fore-thought. The other answers are incorrect interpretations of the text.

19. **(C)** This is most likely taken from a research journal since it is written with a technical focus. It is not written to entertain, so it is not from a novel. It is not likely from a textbook since it is not purely informative in nature.

20. **(A)** The e-mail is definitely written to draw a policy infraction to the attention of the human resources department.

21. **(A)** The author is openly calling a policy infraction to the attention of the human resources director.

22. **(B)** The article is describing holism as care for all aspects of the human condition: mind, body, and spirit.

23. **(D)** a parallelogram

24. **(C)** Page 211

25. **(D)** 28

26. **(B)** 26

27. **(A)** OfficeMax and Staples

28. **(B)** 0663

29. **(A)** A

30. **(A)** Calories 125

31. **(C)** Ken is correct since the person is from Massachusetts and the name does not fit in the letter range for Lucy.

32. **(A)** Lucidity in this sentence means "clarity" rather than the ability to be understood.

33. **(C)** If measured on the graph and compared to dates listed total number of days can be computed.

34. **(D)** approximately 0.5

35. **(C)** 12.5 pounds is more than 10 pounds

36. **(C)** 45° Celsius

37. **(B)** The overall price must include shipping and base price.

38. **(D)** It is under a major section so the introduction is a minor section.

39. **(A)** "Perspectives" is the title of a major section.

40. **(B)** Online library catalogs have all printed materials listed for that library and sometimes even national library listings. The national professional organization might be slanted by a bias about the books to use. The other choices offer limited information.

41. **(B)** In most writings italics are used for emphasis, in this case to emphasize a place.

42. **(A)** In this passage bolding is used to emphasize the tone of the message as a polite invitation rather than a mandatory statement.

43. **(D)** The darkest colors on the map are the areas of highest amounts of precipitation.

44. **(B)** The telephone book entries are in alphabetical order. So the only entry possible is "concession supplies" listed between "comp" and "cont."

45. **(D)** The answer is based on Monday–Friday, and the use of a friend's equipment.

46. **(A)** Advertisements are written to persuade you to purchase a product.

47. **(D)** 2 B is the cruise available during her time off in her cost range.

48. **(B)** Australia is the only one of the countries not in Europe.

Mathematics

1. **(C)** $3+(4\times[5-2])=3+(4\times3)$
$$=3+12$$
$$=15$$
Simplify the expression with the innermost parentheses first. Then solve the next parentheses. $3 + 12 = 15$

2. **(B)** $(3+2)^2-7=5^2-7$
$$=25-7$$
$$=18$$
Simplify the innermost parentheses, after clearing the exponent; thus $25 - 7 = 18$.

3. **(A)** 532
   $\underline{-79}$
   453

   When subtracting whole numbers, numbers are arranged in columns with like place values in each column.

4. **(C)** This option is correct. Thus:

   1,050
   $\underline{-105}$
     945

5. **(B)** Since each tablet is 75 mg, and 225 mg is ordered, there are three sets of 75 in each 225. Therefore the patient should receive $\dfrac{225}{75}$ or 3 tablets.

6. **(C)** $(6+250)\times\$20=256\times\$20=\$5,120.$

7. **(D)** $\dfrac{3}{6}+\dfrac{2}{3}=\dfrac{3\cdot1}{6\cdot1}+\dfrac{2\cdot2}{3\cdot2}=\dfrac{3+4}{6}=\dfrac{7}{6}$

Find the least common denominator. Add the numerators but keep the denominator unchanged.

8. **(B)** $4\dfrac{1}{3}\times\dfrac{6}{3}=\dfrac{13}{3}\times\dfrac{6}{3}=8\dfrac{2}{3}$

or, $4\dfrac{1}{3}\times\dfrac{6}{3}=\dfrac{13}{3}\times\dfrac{6}{3}=\dfrac{13}{1}\times\dfrac{2}{3}=8\dfrac{2}{3}$

9. **(C)** $0.422\times6.13=2.58686$, which simplifies to 2.587

Remove decimals from factors by moving the decimal to the right. In this case, 0.442 has three decimal places and 6.13 has two decimal spaces, which total five decimal places. Count back five decimal places from the end of 258686. The decimal belongs between the 2 and the 5.

10. **(A)** Since 2.6 squared is 6.76, and 2.7 squared is 7.29, the square root of 7 must be right in between 2.6 and 2.7.

11. **(B)** $0.007\times100=0.7\%$.

12. **(C)** The expression 45/625 is converted to a decimal by dividing the dividend 45 by the divisor. The quotient is 0.072.

13. **(B)** Convert each fraction to a common denominator and then rank by largest numerator (largest number). Thus: A $\dfrac{240}{420}$, B $\dfrac{350}{420}$, C $\dfrac{266}{420}$, and D $\dfrac{315}{420}$.

14. **(D)** Since this is an estimate, start with the easiest numbers to divide. B $\dfrac{450,500}{50}=9,010$ which is too high. C 400, $\dfrac{500}{50}=8,010$ which is too low. Since option A is lower still, the only possible option is D.

15. **(C)** $(6,544.25+3,500.50+240.75)-(1,475+2,250)=10,285.50-3,725=\$6,560.50$

16. **(B)** (29.21×36 hours $\times 2$ weeks $= \$2,103.12$ beginning salary) – ($565.13 + 100.22 + 125.15 = \$790.50$ deductions) $= \$1,312.62$ take-home salary.

17. **(A)** Add all purchased items: $\$3.25+\$2.50\ (\$1.25\times2)+\$1.50=\$7.25$

18. **(B)** $(125\times\$30=3,750)+(25\times\$15=375)=\$4,125$.

19. **(D)** Fraction textile $=1-\left(\dfrac{1}{5}+\dfrac{1}{75}+\dfrac{1}{15}\right)$

$=1-\left(\dfrac{15}{75}+\dfrac{1}{75}+\dfrac{5}{75}\right)$

$=1-\dfrac{21}{75}$

$=\dfrac{54}{75}$

20. **(B)** If 12 students make 9% of the class, then the rest of students would make 91% of the class: (91% $\times$ 12 students) divided into 9 = 121 (the rest of the students). Then, 12 (9% of the class) + 121 (91% of the class) = 133 (total number of students).

21. **(A)** 15 males + 106 females = 121 members. 15 males/121 total members = 12.4% of total, and 106 females/121 total members = 87.6%; thus, the ratio of male to female members is 12:88.

22. **(C)** M = 1000, D = 500, C = 100, X = 10, I = 1. Traditionally, the numbers that follow in decreasing number add to the total number. Thus, M = 1000, DC = 600, XI = 11.

23. **(B)** M = 1000, C = 100, X = 10, V = 5, I = 1. If a smaller number is listed before M, L, X, or V, it will be subtracted from the main number. Traditionally, the numbers that follow in decreasing number add to the total number. Thus, M = 1000, C = 100, XC = 90, VIII = 8; which is conventionally written as 1198.

24. **(D)** 1 kilometer = 0.62 miles. Thus, 12 kilometers × 0.62 miles = 7.4 miles.

25. **(B)** 1 fluid ounce = 30 milliliters. So, 270 ml/30 oz. = 9 fluid ounces.

26. **(C)** A yardstick is used for measurements no longer than 1 yard (3 feet or 36 inches).

27. **(A)** (16 inches × 15,000 miles)/1 inch = 240,000 miles.

28. **(B)** The dependent variable is the output based on the input.

29. **(C)** The most frequent number of words in Greek tragedies ranges between 7,000 and 8,000 words.

30. **(C)** In a pie chart, the fraction of the circle that would represent the number of students that made an A on the exam would be 1/8.

31. **(A)** $(2x+3)(4x-5)=(2x)(4x)-(2x)(5)+(3)(4x)-(3)(5)$

$$=8x^2-10x+12x-15$$
$$=8x^2+2x-15$$

32. **(C)** If Marla's age is m (and the sum of their ages is x), and she is five years older than her sister, that means that Marla's sister is five years younger and her age can be expressed as $m-5$. Thus,

$$m+m-5=x$$
$$2m-5=x$$

33. **(B)** $5(3z+2)=6z-8$

$$15z+10-10=6z-8-10$$
$$15z-6z=6z-6z-18$$
$$9z=-18$$
$$z=-\frac{18}{9}$$
$$z=-2$$

34. **(D)** $x-20 > 15$

$$x < -15 + 20 \text{ or } x > 15 + 20$$
$$x < 5 \text{ or } x > 35$$

Since there is a greater than connector, the connecting word is "and."

Science

1. **(B)** Tin has the highest atomic weight of the elements listed.

 2. **(A)** It will have 8 since that is the atomic number. The atomic number is the number of protons.

3. **(B)** The sun always rises in the east no matter the hemisphere.

4. **(B)** Kinetic energy is based on an object's motion. Potential energy is stored.

5. **(B)** An enzyme is a protein catalyst in living organisms.

6. **(A)** If you have an element that has 20 protons, 21 neutrons and 18 electrons, this atom would have a charge of +2. The electronic charge is positive toward the protons since there are more of them than electrons in this element, and an atomic weight of 41 is obtained by adding protons and neutrons. Electrons have very little weight to add to the element.

7. **(D)** The alkali metals have a single valence electron; they want to lose that electron and are most commonly found in the +1 oxidation state. They are very active with a single electron in their outer orbit.

8. **(D)** The scientific notation of the substance is 1×10^{-4}. This can then be converted to a pH by using $pH = -\log (1 \times 10^{-4}) = -(-4) = 4$.

9. **(D)** Saturated hydrocarbons that have single bonds are called alkanes, and they are the most basic structure of hydrocarbon. They have single bonds with carbon.

10. **(B)** Sulfur and oxygen share a double bond and single bond to make the compound.

11. **(B)** What is the balanced equation for

    ___FeS+___O_2 → ___ Fe_2O_3 +____SO_2? Since Fe and S are equal across the formula, begin by balancing the O then adjust the other elements to balance across sides. The first step of balancing O includes finding the common divisor. The divisor must include 2 and 3 to balance the formula. The simplest conversion for both sides of the formula would be 14. With the increase in elements in each O compound, the Fe and S must be increased in the formula to the left to balance.

    $4 FeS + 7 O_2 \rightarrow 2 Fe_2O_3 + 4 SO_2$

12. **(C)** Water is considered the standard for the neutral pH 7.

13. **(B)** Atomic motion is what changes a substance to another state. This can be accomplished with heat change and pressure on the substance.

14. **(D)** Scientific research is important in order to use the information for new applications that may provide a greater standard of living for all.

15. **(D)** This is not stated as a research hypothesis. It is just an interest.

16. **(B)** They are in the process of data collection.

17. **(B)** The "dependent variable" is what is being acted upon; in other words, it is the thing that is influenced by the "independent variable" or the cause of the change.

18. **(A)** Radon is the cause of the possible change in health.

19. **(C)** Qualitative research rarely has the data points preset. The researcher decides when there is enough data as the data is being analyzed.

20. **(C)** When a researcher is exploring an original idea the process is inductive. Deductive reasoning starts at the theory and the research progresses in testing the theory.

21. **(C)** In this study neither the subjects nor the researchers know what intervention is being tested on each individual participant.

22. **(A)** The study has been replicated with the same results.

23. **(C)** An extraneous variable is one that comes about without explanation and can change the results.

24. **(D)** The eukaryotic cell genetic information is in the nucleus.

25. **(A)** One parent has the trait and the other does not. This would allow for a 50% chance that another child of the couple would be affected.

26. **(B)** This is listed from larger to smaller classification.

27. **(B)** Alleles determine mutations in gene structure.

28. **(A)** Uracil is in RNA.

29. **(C)** Mitochondria are in charge of energy production for the cell (ATP).

30. **(A)** Plant cells have large vacuoles to store water.

31. **(D)** The sister chromatids allow for genetic variability. These structures are not present in mitosis so the reproductions are identical.

32. **(D)** Some chemotherapy agents block phases in cell replication.

33. **(D)** They are in the nucleoid body in these bacterial cells.

34. **(B)** RNA translate DNA codes into protein.

35. **(D)** The aging ovaries may allow for mistakes in replicating the fertilized egg, creating an extra Trisomy 21 allele.

36. **(C)** Active acquired immunity results from immunizations.

37. **(A)** Epithelial tissues do not need their own blood supply.

38. **(B)** The nervous system is the body's regulator.

39. **(A)** They bind to a receptor (chemical reaction).

40. **(A)** The medulla controls this function.

41. **(C)** Higher altitudes have fewer atmospheres of pressure so partial pressure of oxygen is lessened.

42. **(C)** Since he smoked for thirty years, it was probably due to the prolonged exposure to carcinogens in smoke.

43. **(C)** The prefrontal lobe controls behavior and organized thinking.

44. **(C)** The left ventricle pushes blood all over the body so the pressure would be higher.

45. **(B)** Oxygenated blood flows through the pulmonary veins, leaving the highly oxygenated area of the lung to provide blood to the body.

46. **(A)** Cardiac muscles are arranged in branching networks.

47. **(D)** Estrogen is the hormone for secondary sex characteristics in women.

48. **(C)** The renal system controls excretion of fluid waste products.

49. **(D)** IgA would most likely be found in saliva.

50. **(B)** Parasympathetic stimulation accomplishes normal digestive function of each system.

51. **(C)** It is converted to conjugated bilirubin.

52. **(B)** This rapid immune response is caused by the histamine release.

53. **(B)** This is the most painful since there are more nerve receptors in this particular layer of skin.

54. **(A)** This baldness is called alopecia.

English and Language Usage

1. **(B)** This option contains the proper verb *spoke* to complete the sentence. The other options are incorrect in either grammar or case.

2. **(C)** This option correctly identifies *John* as a noun and *trip* as an object.

3. **(C)** This option contains correct subject–verb agreement: "club seems" and "everyone gets." All other options contain incorrect subject–verb agreement with regard to number or case.

4. **(D)** This option contains correct subject–verb agreement: "the crowd… cheers." All other options contain incorrect subject–verb agreement with regard to number.

5. **(B)** The antecedent, *Sally*, is singular and feminine, which means that *she* is the only correct answer. All other options are incorrect either in number, gender, or case.

6. **(C)** This option correctly completes the sentence as it contains the correct pronoun to use. All other options are incorrect pronouns to use in this case.

7. **(C)** This option correctly contains double quotation marks around the whole quote. Option D has no quotation marks to properly indicate direct dialogue, and options A and B contain quotations in the wrong places.

8. **(C)** This option correctly contains double quotation marks around the whole quote. Option A unnecessarily adds single quotes, option B contains quotations in the wrong places, and option D has no quotation marks to properly indicate direct dialogue.

9. **(D)** This option is an example of second-person point of view. Option A is an example of third-person point of view. Options B and C are examples of first-person point of view.

10. **(B)** This option is an example of first-person point of view. Options A and D are examples of third-person point of view. Option C is an example of second-person point of view.

11. **(C)** This option effectively uses transitional words to combine the sentences into a single sentence to reflect the original meaning of the group of sentences. All other options may lead to confusion of the writer's original intent.

12. **(A)** This option effectively uses transitional words to combine the sentences into a single sentence that still reflects the original meaning of the group of sentences.

13. **(C)** This option rightly and properly defines the word *vagabond* (which has nothing to do with finances, money loans, or debts). All other options are incorrect.

14. **(B)** This option amply and correctly defines the word *circumspect*. All other options are incorrect.

15. **(C)** The prefix *hyper-* originates from the Greek language. The word *hyperthermia* means "elevated body temperature." Therefore, it can be concluded that this particular patient had symptoms of fever.

16. **(D)** The suffix *-ology* originates from the Greek language. The word *pathophysiology* means "study of diseases." Therefore, it can be concluded that this course was not necessarily about disease prevention.

17. **(C)** This option is the correct spelling. *Accompanied* is a commonly misspelled word: it has two *c*'s and ends in *ed*.

18. **(B)** This option alone is spelled correctly. All other options are spelled incorrectly.

19. **(B)** This option contains the correct word that completes the given sentence. The word ending in "about debt" adds strength to the meaning of *principal*.

20. **(C)** This option contains the only word set that completes the given sentence. *Your* and *you're* are commonly misspelled homophone (sound alike) words.

21. **(D)** This option is spelled correctly; *except* is a commonly misspelled word. The pronoun *these* (other shipmen in the ship) offers a cue to identify *except* as the correctly spelled word.

22. **(A)** This option is spelled correctly. All other options are commonly misspelled words: *genera* (plural of *genus*) is not *genre* (literary category), *stationery* (desk items) is not *stationary* (unmoving, as in bad traffic), and *your* (possessive pronoun) is not *you're* (contraction of *you are*).

23. **(C)** The term *Old South* is properly capitalized, as it refers to a particular historico-geographic region. None of the other options follows correct rules of capitalization.

24. **(D)** The word *Lake* should be capitalized, as it is used as a proper noun in this context. There is no need to capitalize the words in options A, B, or C.

25. **(B)** To correctly punctuate the sentence, a semicolon is required to precede the conjunctive adverbs that connect sentence elements of equal rank: *therefore,* in this case.

26. **(C)** This function alone follows punctuation marks correctly to complete the sentence above. A semicolon may be placed between two related independent clauses.

27. **(C)** This option is constructed as a simple sentence containing one subject and one verb. Although the sentence is detailed, there are no clauses adding to the complexity of the sentence structure, as is the case in option D. Options A and B are not complete sentences.

28. **(D)** This option is constructed as a simple sentence with one subject and a compound verb. Although the sentence is detailed, there are no clauses adding to the complexity of the sentence structure, as in the case of all other options.

29. **(A)** This option makes one clause subordinate to the other by the addition of a subordinating conjunction. Options B and D contain two clauses of equal weight, and option C has opposite focus (on the tourist's amazement rather than on her gazing through the mall).

30. **(B)** This option completes the sentence as a simple sentence. All other options are examples of compound sentences.

31. **(B)** This option clearly and succinctly conveys the writer's intent to accurately describe the event. The other options are written in ways in which the writer's intent might be confused.

32. **(C)** This option is an example of the use of grammar to enhance clarity and readability. The four sentences are combined into one clear, succinct sentence that is easy to read and understand. The other options, while employing correct grammar to condense the four sentences, do not do so in a manner that clearly expresses the writer's intent.

33. **(C)** This option effectively uses transitional words to combine the sentences into a single sentence that still reflects the original meaning of the group of sentences.

34. **(D)** This option effectively uses transitional words to combine the sentences into a single sentence that still reflects the original meaning of the group of sentences.

Practice

TEST 3

ANSWER SHEET
Practice Test 3

PRACTICE TEST 3

READING

1. Ⓐ Ⓑ Ⓒ Ⓓ
2. Ⓐ Ⓑ Ⓒ Ⓓ
3. Ⓐ Ⓑ Ⓒ Ⓓ
4. Ⓐ Ⓑ Ⓒ Ⓓ
5. Ⓐ Ⓑ Ⓒ Ⓓ
6. Ⓐ Ⓑ Ⓒ Ⓓ
7. Ⓐ Ⓑ Ⓒ Ⓓ
8. Ⓐ Ⓑ Ⓒ Ⓓ
9. Ⓐ Ⓑ Ⓒ Ⓓ
10. Ⓐ Ⓑ Ⓒ Ⓓ
11. Ⓐ Ⓑ Ⓒ Ⓓ
12. Ⓐ Ⓑ Ⓒ Ⓓ

13. Ⓐ Ⓑ Ⓒ Ⓓ
14. Ⓐ Ⓑ Ⓒ Ⓓ
15. Ⓐ Ⓑ Ⓒ Ⓓ
16. Ⓐ Ⓑ Ⓒ Ⓓ
17. Ⓐ Ⓑ Ⓒ Ⓓ
18. Ⓐ Ⓑ Ⓒ Ⓓ
19. Ⓐ Ⓑ Ⓒ Ⓓ
20. Ⓐ Ⓑ Ⓒ Ⓓ
21. Ⓐ Ⓑ Ⓒ Ⓓ
22. Ⓐ Ⓑ Ⓒ Ⓓ
23. Ⓐ Ⓑ Ⓒ Ⓓ
24. Ⓐ Ⓑ Ⓒ Ⓓ

25. Ⓐ Ⓑ Ⓒ Ⓓ
26. Ⓐ Ⓑ Ⓒ Ⓓ
27. Ⓐ Ⓑ Ⓒ Ⓓ
28. Ⓐ Ⓑ Ⓒ Ⓓ
29. Ⓐ Ⓑ Ⓒ Ⓓ
30. Ⓐ Ⓑ Ⓒ Ⓓ
31. Ⓐ Ⓑ Ⓒ Ⓓ
32. Ⓐ Ⓑ Ⓒ Ⓓ
33. Ⓐ Ⓑ Ⓒ Ⓓ
34. Ⓐ Ⓑ Ⓒ Ⓓ
35. Ⓐ Ⓑ Ⓒ Ⓓ
36. Ⓐ Ⓑ Ⓒ Ⓓ

37. Ⓐ Ⓑ Ⓒ Ⓓ
38. Ⓐ Ⓑ Ⓒ Ⓓ
39. Ⓐ Ⓑ Ⓒ Ⓓ
40. Ⓐ Ⓑ Ⓒ Ⓓ
41. Ⓐ Ⓑ Ⓒ Ⓓ
42. Ⓐ Ⓑ Ⓒ Ⓓ
43. Ⓐ Ⓑ Ⓒ Ⓓ
44. Ⓐ Ⓑ Ⓒ Ⓓ
45. Ⓐ Ⓑ Ⓒ Ⓓ
46. Ⓐ Ⓑ Ⓒ Ⓓ
47. Ⓐ Ⓑ Ⓒ Ⓓ
48. Ⓐ Ⓑ Ⓒ Ⓓ

MATHEMATICS

1. Ⓐ Ⓑ Ⓒ Ⓓ
2. Ⓐ Ⓑ Ⓒ Ⓓ
3. Ⓐ Ⓑ Ⓒ Ⓓ
4. Ⓐ Ⓑ Ⓒ Ⓓ
5. Ⓐ Ⓑ Ⓒ Ⓓ
6. Ⓐ Ⓑ Ⓒ Ⓓ
7. Ⓐ Ⓑ Ⓒ Ⓓ
8. Ⓐ Ⓑ Ⓒ Ⓓ
9. Ⓐ Ⓑ Ⓒ Ⓓ

10. Ⓐ Ⓑ Ⓒ Ⓓ
11. Ⓐ Ⓑ Ⓒ Ⓓ
12. Ⓐ Ⓑ Ⓒ Ⓓ
13. Ⓐ Ⓑ Ⓒ Ⓓ
14. Ⓐ Ⓑ Ⓒ Ⓓ
15. Ⓐ Ⓑ Ⓒ Ⓓ
16. Ⓐ Ⓑ Ⓒ Ⓓ
17. Ⓐ Ⓑ Ⓒ Ⓓ
18. Ⓐ Ⓑ Ⓒ Ⓓ

19. Ⓐ Ⓑ Ⓒ Ⓓ
20. Ⓐ Ⓑ Ⓒ Ⓓ
21. Ⓐ Ⓑ Ⓒ Ⓓ
22. Ⓐ Ⓑ Ⓒ Ⓓ
23. Ⓐ Ⓑ Ⓒ Ⓓ
24. Ⓐ Ⓑ Ⓒ Ⓓ
25. Ⓐ Ⓑ Ⓒ Ⓓ
26. Ⓐ Ⓑ Ⓒ Ⓓ
27. Ⓐ Ⓑ Ⓒ Ⓓ

28. Ⓐ Ⓑ Ⓒ Ⓓ
29. Ⓐ Ⓑ Ⓒ Ⓓ
30. Ⓐ Ⓑ Ⓒ Ⓓ
31. Ⓐ Ⓑ Ⓒ Ⓓ
32. Ⓐ Ⓑ Ⓒ Ⓓ
33. Ⓐ Ⓑ Ⓒ Ⓓ
34. Ⓐ Ⓑ Ⓒ Ⓓ

SCIENCE

1. Ⓐ Ⓑ Ⓒ Ⓓ	15. Ⓐ Ⓑ Ⓒ Ⓓ	29. Ⓐ Ⓑ Ⓒ Ⓓ	43. Ⓐ Ⓑ Ⓒ Ⓓ
2. Ⓐ Ⓑ Ⓒ Ⓓ	16. Ⓐ Ⓑ Ⓒ Ⓓ	30. Ⓐ Ⓑ Ⓒ Ⓓ	44. Ⓐ Ⓑ Ⓒ Ⓓ
3. Ⓐ Ⓑ Ⓒ Ⓓ	17. Ⓐ Ⓑ Ⓒ Ⓓ	31. Ⓐ Ⓑ Ⓒ Ⓓ	45. Ⓐ Ⓑ Ⓒ Ⓓ
4. Ⓐ Ⓑ Ⓒ Ⓓ	18. Ⓐ Ⓑ Ⓒ Ⓓ	32. Ⓐ Ⓑ Ⓒ Ⓓ	46. Ⓐ Ⓑ Ⓒ Ⓓ
5. Ⓐ Ⓑ Ⓒ Ⓓ	19. Ⓐ Ⓑ Ⓒ Ⓓ	33. Ⓐ Ⓑ Ⓒ Ⓓ	47. Ⓐ Ⓑ Ⓒ Ⓓ
6. Ⓐ Ⓑ Ⓒ Ⓓ	20. Ⓐ Ⓑ Ⓒ Ⓓ	34. Ⓐ Ⓑ Ⓒ Ⓓ	48. Ⓐ Ⓑ Ⓒ Ⓓ
7. Ⓐ Ⓑ Ⓒ Ⓓ	21. Ⓐ Ⓑ Ⓒ Ⓓ	35. Ⓐ Ⓑ Ⓒ Ⓓ	49. Ⓐ Ⓑ Ⓒ Ⓓ
8. Ⓐ Ⓑ Ⓒ Ⓓ	22. Ⓐ Ⓑ Ⓒ Ⓓ	36. Ⓐ Ⓑ Ⓒ Ⓓ	50. Ⓐ Ⓑ Ⓒ Ⓓ
9. Ⓐ Ⓑ Ⓒ Ⓓ	23. Ⓐ Ⓑ Ⓒ Ⓓ	37. Ⓐ Ⓑ Ⓒ Ⓓ	51. Ⓐ Ⓑ Ⓒ Ⓓ
10. Ⓐ Ⓑ Ⓒ Ⓓ	24. Ⓐ Ⓑ Ⓒ Ⓓ	38. Ⓐ Ⓑ Ⓒ Ⓓ	52. Ⓐ Ⓑ Ⓒ Ⓓ
11. Ⓐ Ⓑ Ⓒ Ⓓ	25. Ⓐ Ⓑ Ⓒ Ⓓ	39. Ⓐ Ⓑ Ⓒ Ⓓ	53. Ⓐ Ⓑ Ⓒ Ⓓ
12. Ⓐ Ⓑ Ⓒ Ⓓ	26. Ⓐ Ⓑ Ⓒ Ⓓ	40. Ⓐ Ⓑ Ⓒ Ⓓ	54. Ⓐ Ⓑ Ⓒ Ⓓ
13. Ⓐ Ⓑ Ⓒ Ⓓ	27. Ⓐ Ⓑ Ⓒ Ⓓ	41. Ⓐ Ⓑ Ⓒ Ⓓ	
14. Ⓐ Ⓑ Ⓒ Ⓓ	28. Ⓐ Ⓑ Ⓒ Ⓓ	42. Ⓐ Ⓑ Ⓒ Ⓓ	

ENGLISH AND LANGUAGE USAGE

1. Ⓐ Ⓑ Ⓒ Ⓓ	10. Ⓐ Ⓑ Ⓒ Ⓓ	19. Ⓐ Ⓑ Ⓒ Ⓓ	28. Ⓐ Ⓑ Ⓒ Ⓓ
2. Ⓐ Ⓑ Ⓒ Ⓓ	11. Ⓐ Ⓑ Ⓒ Ⓓ	20. Ⓐ Ⓑ Ⓒ Ⓓ	29. Ⓐ Ⓑ Ⓒ Ⓓ
3. Ⓐ Ⓑ Ⓒ Ⓓ	12. Ⓐ Ⓑ Ⓒ Ⓓ	21. Ⓐ Ⓑ Ⓒ Ⓓ	30. Ⓐ Ⓑ Ⓒ Ⓓ
4. Ⓐ Ⓑ Ⓒ Ⓓ	13. Ⓐ Ⓑ Ⓒ Ⓓ	22. Ⓐ Ⓑ Ⓒ Ⓓ	31. Ⓐ Ⓑ Ⓒ Ⓓ
5. Ⓐ Ⓑ Ⓒ Ⓓ	14. Ⓐ Ⓑ Ⓒ Ⓓ	23. Ⓐ Ⓑ Ⓒ Ⓓ	32. Ⓐ Ⓑ Ⓒ Ⓓ
6. Ⓐ Ⓑ Ⓒ Ⓓ	15. Ⓐ Ⓑ Ⓒ Ⓓ	24. Ⓐ Ⓑ Ⓒ Ⓓ	33. Ⓐ Ⓑ Ⓒ Ⓓ
7. Ⓐ Ⓑ Ⓒ Ⓓ	16. Ⓐ Ⓑ Ⓒ Ⓓ	25. Ⓐ Ⓑ Ⓒ Ⓓ	34. Ⓐ Ⓑ Ⓒ Ⓓ
8. Ⓐ Ⓑ Ⓒ Ⓓ	17. Ⓐ Ⓑ Ⓒ Ⓓ	26. Ⓐ Ⓑ Ⓒ Ⓓ	
9. Ⓐ Ⓑ Ⓒ Ⓓ	18. Ⓐ Ⓑ Ⓒ Ⓓ	27. Ⓐ Ⓑ Ⓒ Ⓓ	

Part 1: Reading

Time: 58 minutes

48 questions

QUESTIONS 1 THROUGH 6 ARE BASED ON THE FOLLOWING PASSAGE.

Morning Break

Often break is enjoyed by all in the company. This morning is different. One person is absent. We don't know why she left, but the effect was severe. Her departure left all without a reason to walk down the hall to see the sunshine emanating from her desk. She added life to the common everyday office experience. There was always a sarcastic retort whenever the boss walked by. She needed an early morning report of a positive 'whale' sign and then would remark "too bad" if it was positive.

The triangulation potentials were high and we did succumb to the temptation. To be able to talk openly about someone else is stimulating. It does take away from the possibility of direct communication, though. She would keep all of our confidences and support us during hard times.

Since she left, we have to talk to each person directly if we feel bad on any particular day when she is not here. This communication adds to the overall camaraderie of the work place. I am hoping to have break with someone new today and make a new connection. I guess the real 'whale' has left the building, but the boss remains. Morning break could be a wonderful experience today!

1. In the title "Morning Break," how does the title relate to the overall passage content?

    (A) why breaks are important
    (B) how daily activities should be controlled by break time
    (C) how break-time communication can change the workplace
    (D) how to schedule breaks to encourage communication

2. Identify the purpose of this quotation from the passage: "I am hoping to have morning break with someone new today."

    (A) to explain the topic
    (B) to continue the narrative
    (C) to persuade the reader
    (D) to provide precise information

3. What was this passage communicating to the reader?

   (A) Things are better if discussed in private.
   (B) Morning breaks should be solitary events.
   (C) Direct communication is best.
   (D) Whales should not have breaks.

4. What was the author's bias about communication in the above passage?

   (A) It should be fun even if painful to some.
   (B) It should be closed.
   (C) It should be without triangulation.
   (D) It should be severe.

5. What is an example of cause and effect structure in the passage above?

   (A) To be able to talk openly about someone else is stimulating.
   (B) When one person is absent the others act differently.
   (C) Morning break could be a wonderful experience today!
   (D) She would keep all of our confidences and support us during hard times.

6. Which of these statements is an example of the writer's failed logic regarding communication at the workplace?

   (A) puzzlement about the situation
   (B) the communication will never improve
   (C) one person seemed essential to the fun
   (D) communication should be direct

QUESTIONS 7 THROUGH 11 ARE BASED ON THE FOLLOWING PASSAGE.

Learning How to Think

If you consider how we think, you might consider it to be partial or haphazard. Can we learn how to think with sufficient quality or quantity to sustain us in today's complex society? An organized way of thinking must be developed to direct our lives into clarity and direction. This ability is way beyond common sense or the ability to function today. It is a way of thinking about how you are thinking as a self-direction toward an acceptable intellectual standard of thought. Beyond the scientific method, an effective process will lead to accuracy and precision of thought toward a significance of living.

People who have attained this level of thought know that there is purpose for reasoning. The correct frame of thought described by scholars enables a basis in evidence-based life far above the mundane. All thought has reasons, implications, and consequences. It is rare for a thoughtful person to become lost in a story or fail to gain significance from a conversation. This skill may be practiced and learned with a specific concentration on what you are thinking. Think about how you are thinking and move beyond the mundane!

7. The last sentence in the passage summarizes the author's overall intent. Why was this passage written?

   (A) for the purpose of entertainment
   (B) to evoke emotion
   (C) to present some fact of interest
   (D) to sway the reader to a particular viewpoint

8. Under which heading in a textbook would this passage most logically belong?

   (A) Introduction
   (B) Reasons for thinking well
   (C) Critical thinking while studying
   (D) How to determine if you are thinking well

9. On which type of website would this passage most likely be found?

   (A) news site
   (B) government site
   (C) historical site
   (D) organizational site

10. Which phrase from the passage above demonstrates a description?

    (A) It is rare for a thoughtful person to become lost in a story or fail to gain significance from a conversation.
    (B) If you consider how we think, you might consider it to be partial or haphazard.
    (C) Can we learn how to think with sufficient quality or quantity to sustain us in today's complex society?
    (D) An organized way of thinking must be developed to direct our lives into clarity and direction.

11. "An organized way of thinking must be developed to direct our lives into clarity and direction." Which term below best describes the content of this quote?

    (A) topic
    (B) supporting detail
    (C) main idea
    (D) theme

Universal beginnings and endings have their place in everyday activities. We usually start each activity with an action that will be repeated before any other action. Introducing yourself before an interaction and summarizing the conversation is how we expect an interaction to unfold.

12. Based on the passage above, what is the author's overall conclusion regarding universal beginnings and endings?

    (A) They will always vary slightly.
    (B) They will allow for consistency in how we interact.
    (C) The activity is not worth the effort.
    (D) We should not expect these to be used at all.

Video streaming is becoming a replacement for traditional television. The new companies are offering series and movies for a nominal charge much less than cable television services. There are over 200 channels available for cable viewers to watch: that simply is not what viewers want to see. Video streaming companies provide what viewers want, when they want it, and offer a choice of devices to watch on.

13. Who is the intended audience of the above passage?

    (A) people who frequent movie theaters

    (B) cable subscribers

    (C) computer users

    (D) video streamers

Get tighter abdominal muscles with the abdominal exerciser. This new device will slim your abdominal area and tighten the abdominal muscles without horrible exercises. This device will trim you while you work as usual during your day… no matter your activity level.

14. What is the false assumption used to convince the reader in the above advertisement?

    (A) The exerciser will tighten all abdominal muscles.

    (B) Tighter abdominal muscles means weight loss.

    (C) Muscles need exercising.

    (D) Daily activity will not trim the abdominal area.

Make more than your share of Social Security monthly benefits. There is a way to 'beat the system' and receive up to one thousand dollars a month more than you are now. Sign up for the free information booklet, and get the guidance you need to help you make more.

15. What is the implied message to the reader in the above passage?

    (A) There is not enough money to pay anyone extra.

    (B) There is a way to fool the government.

    (C) More money will not be available.

    (D) Act fast so the author can help you.

Keeping your car running is challenging during cold weather. It involves some in-depth diagnostic approaches to be successful. In winter, it is especially important to check the anti-freeze in the radiator, the windshield washer solution, and the tire pressure to ensure safe running of your vehicle during colder weather. If your service professional does not complete these basic checks, you could be stranded with a vehicle that is non-functional. These checks are easily done by the owner and would be best done by someone that has a vested interest in the operation of the vehicle.

16. What should the reader learn about car care from the above passage?

    (A) to do car care without preparation

    (B) to attempt advanced auto service

    (C) some auto service can be done by the owner

    (D) some auto care is needed in the summer

The group had assembled for graduation. The candidates were excited and walked proudly. We were all puzzled by the presence of one of the participants who had not completed all requirements for graduation. We remained silent. There was no official graduate document being presented, so no harm done. The "graduate" told us through social media that he was counseled the following week. We were concerned that the graduation was allowed to happen even though counseling occurred. We felt angry since we had done the work to finish our studies and the "graduate" had not.

17. We felt angry since we had done the work to finish our studies and the "graduate" had not." What is the group communicating by this statement?

    (A) humor
    (B) information
    (C) a convincing argument
    (D) emotion

Researchers of our time believe that investigators should merely record scientific information and not explore cause and effect. The fullest understanding of a thing is interpretation of the facts; not just fulfillment of a wish.

18. Which type of literature is the above passage most likely from?

    (A) textbook
    (B) science fiction novel
    (C) research journal
    (D) mystery novel

As all sat around the campfire, each person interpreted a sound heard. The imaginations flew into each person's sensitivity so that while the stories became more extreme each thought froze in the air. The participants expressed the need to stop the stories, but they continued until everyone was extremely cold and the campfire burned down.

19. Which type of literature is the above passage most likely from?

    (A) textbook
    (B) science fiction novel
    (C) research journal
    (D) mystery novel

QUESTIONS 20 AND 21 ARE BASED ON THE FOLLOWING E-MAIL WHICH WAS SENT TO A CUSTOMER.

Susan,

We have found a great savings opportunity for you. Purchase your insurance in a package to save cash now. If you combine auto and home coverage, you'll no longer have to worry about protecting your belongings, plus you could end up saving up to $350 per year! Please contact me today.

Thank you,

Juan Ball

360–452-6666

Allied Insurance Group

---

20. What is the main purpose of this e-mail?

   (A) The author wants to increase the customer's insurance coverage.
   (B) The author wants to offer a discount in price.
   (C) The author disagrees with the way that the customer pays.
   (D) The author wants to chat about insurance.

21. What is the author's bias regarding the option mentioned in the e-mail?

   (A) It is best to have insurance in separate packages.
   (B) It is difficult to identify the author's bias.
   (C) Bundling is best.
   (D) There are no biases noted.

I would like to **stress** the need to approach the dog with caution. He is likely to pull you down or push you over because of his size.

22. What is the meaning of *stress* in the passage above?

   (A) be fearful
   (B) to pronounce the word with emphasis
   (C) be worried
   (D) to emphasize a fact

23. Based on the compass and key in the map below, determine your location after following the driving directions.

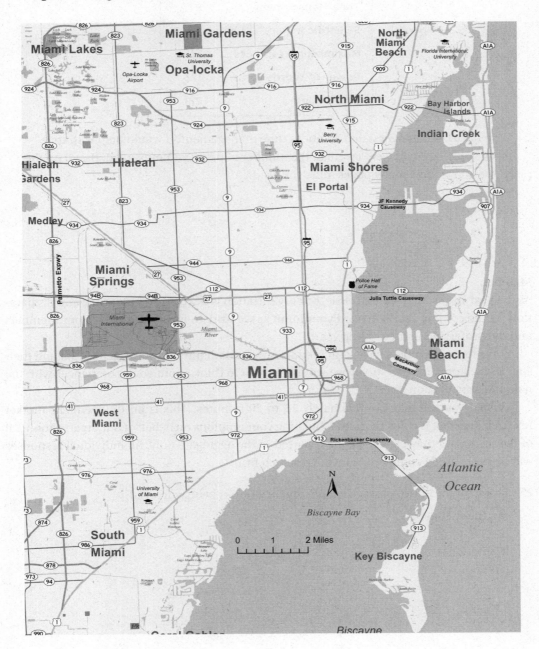

Step 1. Depart from intersection of 826 and 836.

Step 2. Travel 4.5 miles north and turn southeast.

Step 3. Travel 5 miles and turn east, and then travel 4.5 miles.

Where are you?

(A) Police Hall of Fame

(B) Miami Beach

(C) Florida International University

(D) heading toward JFK Causeway

Self-awareness	55
Time Management	87
Scientific Inquiry	113
Maximizing Resources	143
Power of Words	173
Test Taking	221

24. You have been assigned to read about time management. It would help with time management if you were aware of the number of pages you must read. Based on the table above, how many pages must you read?

(A) 22

(B) 25

(C) 28

(D) 30

Member,

As the year begins to draw to a close, our organization is deep into its planning and preparation for the coming year. We need your input as we work to meet the needs of our members and the profession in the coming year.

While many members have joint membership in both the national organization and their state association, for this survey we would like you to think about your experiences with the national organization only.

This survey will take approximately 15 to 20 minutes. This is an independent market research firm that is collecting and tabulating your opinions on behalf of our organization. All of the responses they collect will be reported in the aggregate only. All individual responses will be kept strictly confidential by the research firm.

25. Based on the above passage, which organization is being surveyed?

(A) independent

(B) joint

(C) national

(D) state

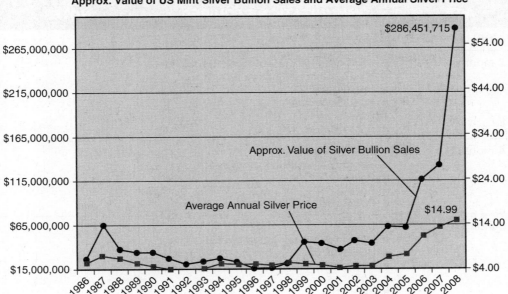

Approx. Value of US Mint Silver Bullion Sales and Average Annual Silver Price

26. Based on the above graph, which year was silver's price most closely aligned with silver's value?

(A) 1994

(B) 1996

(C) 1998

(D) 2000

AGE	IMMUNIZATION REQUIRED	NOTES
Birth	Hepatitis B	
2 months	■ Diptheria, tetanus and pertussis DTaP ■ Haemophilus influenza type b ■ Hepatitis B ■ Pneumococcal ■ Polio ■ Rotavirus	
4 months	■ DTaP ■ Haemophilus influenza type b ■ Pneumococcal ■ Polio ■ Rotavirus	
6 months	■ DTaP ■ Haemophilus influenza type b ■ Hepatitis B ■ Pneumococcal ■ Polio ■ Rotavirus	
6 months and older	Flu	
12 months	■ Chicken Pox (Varicella) ■ DTaP ■ Haemophilus influenza type b ■ Hepatitis A ■ Measles, Mumps, Rubella (MMR) ■ Pneumococcal	
15 months	DTaP	
18 months	Hepatitis A	
4 years	■ Chicken Pox (Varicella) ■ DTaP ■ MMR ■ Polio	
11 years and older	■ Human papillomavirus ■ Meningococcal ■ TDaP	
Special Immunizations 2 years and older	■ Hepatitis A ■ Pneumococcal ■ Meningococcal	Child may need if has: ■ sickle cell disease ■ a damaged spleen ■ immune deficiency ■ chronic disease

27. A four-year-old child with a chronic disease needs age appropriate immunizations. According to table, which combination of immunizations will this child need for this physician office visit?

(A) Chicken Pox (Varicella), DTaP, Haemophilus influenza type b, MMR
(B) Chicken Pox (Varicella), DTaP, MMR, Polio, Meningococcal
(C) Haemophilus influenza type b, Hepatitis B
(D) Human papillomavirus, Meningococcal, TDaP

28. On which page of the yellow pages phone directory would you expect to find phone numbers for "local elementary schools"?

(A) between page headers "egg farm" and "ekg technical schools"
(B) between page headers "electrical contractors" and "engraving"
(C) between page headers "embroidery" and "employment agencies"
(D) between page headers "engineering firms" and "equipment rentals"

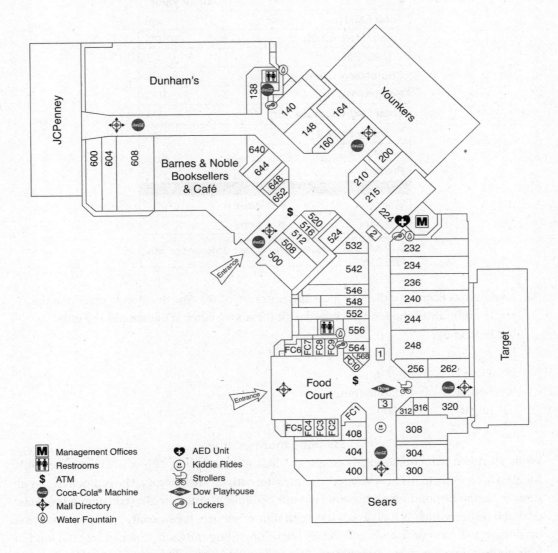

29. A customer has collapsed in front of Sears. According to the above map, where is the closest AED Unit in this mall?

(A) between the Target and Younkers stores
(B) in front of Dunhams
(C) in the food court
(D) in the store at 644 location

Nutrition Facts

Serving Size ½ cup (124 g)
Servings Per Container About 3

Amount Per Serving

Calories 110	Calories from Fat 0

	% Daily Value*
Total Fat 0 g	0%
Saturated Fat 0 g	0%
Trans Fat 0	
Cholesterol 0 mg	0%
Sodium 470 mg	19%
Total Carbohydrate 22 g	7%
Dietary Fiber 8 g	32%
Sugars 2 g	
Protein 7 g	

Vitamin A	0%	●	Vitamin C	0%
Calcium	4%	●	Iron	10%

*Percent Daily Values are based on a 2,000 calorie diet.
Your daily values may be higher or lower depending on your
calorie needs.

30. A woman is keeping a diary of food and nutrient intake. She decided to consume the entire contents of the food packaged with the above label. What should she enter on her food diary?

(A) Calories   250
(B) Fiber   24 grams
(C) Sodium   470 milligrams
(D) Sugar   8 grams

Planning Your Wedding

While sit-down five-course meals create an elegant setting, they can easily break the bank. Meet with caterers to discuss budget-friendly alternatives, such as an all hors d'oeuvres or all dessert buffet. Depending on the time of your ceremony, you may also consider a breakfast or lunch buffet, which usually costs less than dinner service. If you really have your heart set on dinner, talk to your friends and family about providing the food. You can buy the food in bulk at discount club stores and rent chafing and serving dishes from party rental businesses. Some couples with casual, backyard affairs will ask each guest to bring a dish.

31. According to the website advice above, which approach would be the most expensive option for a wedding party?

(A) lunch buffet
(B) dinner meal
(C) all hors d'oeuvres
(D) catered breakfast

32. "The student demonstrated **virtuosity** in his presentation." Which of the following is the best definition of the bolded word?

    (A) clarity
    (B) indecisiveness
    (C) lightheartedness
    (D) exceptional skill

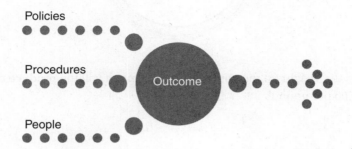

33. The above diagram was presented to a group to allow for open discussion of requirements for success. Which part of the diagram is reflective of resources needed to attain the outcome?

    (A) outcome
    (B) policies
    (C) people
    (D) procedures

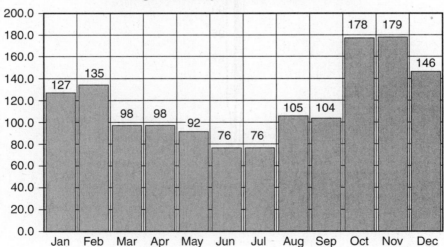

34. According to the graph, the new resident of this region would expect which month to be the driest?

    (A) March
    (B) June
    (C) August
    (D) October

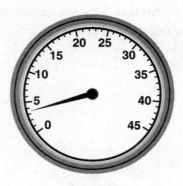

35. According to the weight on the above scale, how much will the produce cost if it is priced at $2.00 per pound?

(A) $5
(B) $6
(C) $7
(D) $8

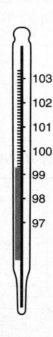

36. Read the current temperature on the thermometer in degrees Fahrenheit.

(A) 98.6°
(B) 99.4°
(C) 100.6°
(D) 103°

University Cost Comparison

UNIVERSITY	TOTAL COST 2010	TOTAL COST 2009	INCREASE
Amherst College	$50,230	$48,352	3.90%
Babson College	$50,866	$48,450	5.00%
Bard College	$51,240	$48,880	4.80%
Bard College at Simon's Rock	$50,775	$49,385	2.80%
Barnard College	$51,976	$49,174	5.70%
Bennington College	$51,950	$49,155	5.70%
Boston College	$52,060	$48,384	7.60%
Bowdoin College	$50,570	$48,260	4.80%
Brandeis University	$50,148	$47,310	6.00%
Brown University	$50,560	$48,660	3.90%
Bryn Mawr College	$50,060	$47,674	5.00%
Bucknell University	$50,250	$47,936	4.80%
California Institute of the Arts	$49,182	$46,838	5.00%

37. According to the table, which university reported the greatest increase in costs between 2009 and 2010?

    (A) Amherst College
    (B) Boston College
    (C) Bucknell University
    (D) California Institute of the Arts

1. Everyday Learning

   A Reading strategies

   B Learning styles

   C How to remember facts

2. During the Test

   A Dealing with anxiety

   B Test-taking strategies for multiple choice tests

   C Test-taking strategies for essay tests

3. After the Test

   A Tips to improve your scores in next test

   B Learning from your patterns

38. Identify the major section dealing with preparing for an exam.

   (A) Everyday Learning
   (B) How to remember facts
   (C) Dealing with anxiety
   (D) Learning from your patterns

39. Identify the minor section that explains how to answer specific test items.

   (A) Everyday Learning
   (B) Learning style
   (C) Test-taking strategies for multiple choice tests
   (D) Tips to improve your scores in next test

40. A person is complaining of low back pain. What would be the best source of information for therapies for pain relief?

   (A) online search
   (B) National Institute of Health
   (C) pharmaceutical web page
   (D) back-pain relief mattress distributor

Customer,

Once your shipment has arrived refer to the Self Installation Guide for easy-to-follow instructions on how to successfully install your telephone upgrade. Make sure you "test" the system according to the instructions before you attempt to troubleshoot the system.

---

41. In the above passage, what is the reason for the hyphens between the words *easy-to-follow?*

 (A) used when writing compound words
 (B) to draw attention to the phrase
 (C) to identify modifiers
 (D) to denote the ending of the story

42. What is the meaning of the quotation marks in the passage?

 (A) to denote the beginning and end of a statement
 (B) to draw attention to the passage
 (C) to identify an opinion
 (D) to add emphasis to the word

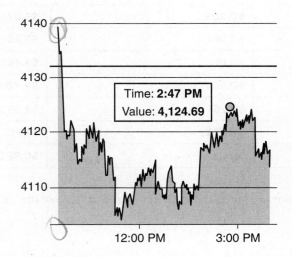

43. According to the graph, what time of day is the highest value trading done in the stock exchange?

 (A) early morning
 (B) noon
 (C) mid-afternoon
 (D) closing

44. The guide words at the top of the page in a phone directory are "recreational vehicles" and "rental cars." What other business could be found on that page?

(A) restaurant supplies
(B) resale shops
(C) recycling center
(D) realtors

Food Cost Comparison

	JANUARY 1913	JANUARY 2013
Bread	$0.056	$1.422
Flour	$0.033	$0.524
Fresh milk, per gallon	$0.089/quart (or 0.356/gallon)	$3.526
Cheese	$0.222	$5.832
Butter	$0.409	$3.501
Coffee	$0.299	$5.902
Potatoes	$0.016	$0.627
Rice	$0.086	$0.715
Sirloin steak	$0.238	$5.705
Round Steak	$0.205	$5.074
Chuck roast	$0.149	$3.696
Pork chops	$0.187	$3.465
Bacon	$0.254	$4.407
Ham	$0.251	$2.693
Eggs, per dozen	$0.373	$1.933
Sugar	$0.058	$0.683

45. Based the table above, which food item has increased in cost the most over the last 100 years?

(A) cheese
(B) flour
(C) milk
(D) sirloin steak

The aurora borealis will dip further south because of a large solar flare that attacked the electromagnetic field of the earth this week. The beautiful phenomenon will be visible as far south as Colorado in the United States.

46. What is the purpose of the above passage?

    (A) to persuade
    (B) to inform
    (C) to entertain
    (D) express feelings

47. This company fulfills a unique, catchall need of several of our clients in the form of all-encompassing marketing materials management. Utilizing our own storage facilities and internal human capital, we take ownership of the shipping logistics, routing, and maintenance of marketing crates, collateral, and event supplies. Alongside meeting management, sourcing, and onsite and virtual placement, we are our client's events deliverables way station.

    What is the primary product being sold in the paragraph above?

    (A) marketing
    (B) materials
    (C) moving
    (D) event management

Chapter 3: Animals of Asia

A Variations

B Location of animal variations

    a. China

    b. India

    c. Japan

    d. Mongolia

    e. New Zealand

48. Based on the pattern in the outline above, which entry doesn't seem to belong?

    (A) India
    (B) Japan
    (C) Mongolia
    (D) New Zealand

Part 2: Mathematics

Time: 51 minutes

34 questions

1. Simplify the expression: $(9-2)^2 - 7$.

    (A) 63
    (B) 36
    (C) 24
    (D) 42

2. Simplify the expression: $9 \times 4 \div 6 \times 3$.

    (A) 2
    (B) 4
    (C) 6
    (D) 8

3. Subtract 1.25 from 0.45.

    (A) 800
    (B) − 0.8
    (C) − 85
    (D) 0.25

4. Take 2,635 from 4,315.

    (A) 6,950
    (B) 1,680
    (C) 1,860
    (D) 2,120

5. If $1,525,250 is the total income expected by a company for the year, and the total expenses listed in the annual budget were $754,025, how much profit would the company expect to make?

    (A) $771,225
    (B) $1,021,135
    (C) $540,125
    (D) $635,535

6. A nurse is to give 65 milligrams (mg) of a certain sedative to a patient. The drug is supplied in 130 mg tablets. How many tablets should this patient receive?

(A) $2\frac{1}{2}$ tablets

(B) 2 tablets

(C) $\frac{1}{2}$ tablet

(D) $1\frac{1}{2}$ tablets

7. Compute the difference: $4\frac{2}{3}-3$.

(A) $\frac{1}{6}$

(B) $\frac{3}{5}$

(C) $\frac{5}{9}$

(D) $\frac{5}{3}$

8. What is the quotient of $\frac{8}{3}\div\frac{6}{5}$?

(A) 20.18

(B) 2.2

(C) 1.2

(D) 8.6

9. Divide 0.034 by 0.465.

(A) 0.073

(B) 0.080

(C) 1.367

(D) 13.68

10. What irrational number can be approximated by 5.1962?

(A) square root of 21

(B) square root of 36

(C) square root of 25

(D) square root of 27

11. 15% of what number is 15?

(A) 150

(B) 100

(C) 125

(D) 200

12. Which of the following fractions is equivalent to the expression 0.025?

(A) $\dfrac{1}{4}$

(B) $\dfrac{1}{40}$

(C) $\dfrac{1}{25}$

(D) $\dfrac{1}{20}$

13. Which of the following numbers is greater?

(A) 0.665

(B) 0.559

(C) 0.661

(D) 0.663

14. Estimate the quotient of: 87,699 ÷ 4,651.

(A) 20.910

(B) 19.011

(C) 18.856

(D) 18.512

15. Reconcile the savings account for this month. The previous balance was $7,453.21. Deposits were made for $2,225.50 and $82.13; interest earned is $2.98, and withdrawals were made for $300, $500, and $1,500. What is the balance after reconciling this account?

(A) $8,865.12

(B) $7,463.82

(C) $6,545.26

(D) $9,678.71

16. An employee's take home pay is $3,125.25 each month. Monthly expenses include: rent $750, food $350.25, utilities $150.24, transportation $150.19. How much does the employee have left from the monthly income?

(A) $1,724.57

(B) $2,551.23

(C) $1,053.21

(D) $1,954.75

17. A customer purchases the following items in a grocery store: 2 yogurt containers for $5 each, 1 pound of bacon for $3.50, 1 loaf of bread for $1.50, 1 pound of coffee for $6.50, and 1 dozen eggs for $2. What is the total cost of groceries before tax?

(A) $18.50

(B) $19.25

(C) $25.75

(D) $23.50

18. A school is planning a nursing graduates pinning ceremony, and 50 students with 20 guests are expected to attend. Each student will receive a pin, and a commemorative lamp; each guest will receive an appreciation certificate. The supply company charges $4.40 for pins, $6.50 for lamps, and $7 for appreciation certificates. What is the total cost for this ceremony?

(A) $895
(B) $358
(C) $685
(D) $583

19. A customer bought several items totaling $654.19 before taxes. How much tax will this customer pay if the tax is 0.073 per dollar?

(A) $61.42
(B) $59.42
(C) $47.76
(D) $42.50

20. On first class day, 5 students out of a total of 35 arrived late. What percent of the students were late to class?

(A) 15.6%
(B) 14.3%
(C) 13.5%
(D) 17.5%

21. Matt travels 160 miles in 3 hours. How far would he travel in 7 hours?

(A) 373.3 miles
(B) 210.1 miles
(C) 320.9 miles
(D) 480.2 miles

22. A diving team found an artifact conspicuously inscribed with the Roman number DCLXXXIV. How is this written in conventional numbers?

(A) 538
(B) 659
(C) 594
(D) 684

23. An artist was designing an Olympic trophy that was to be dated 2014. How is this date written in Roman numerals?

(A) XX-XIV
(B) MMIV
(C) MMXIV
(D) MMXVI

24. How many inches are in 257 centimeters?

(A) 85.28
(B) 101.2
(C) 95.17
(D) 100.8

25. To assist in rehydration, a patient was told to drink 5 quarts of spring water. How many cups would the patient drink?

(A) 25
(B) 15
(C) 12
(D) 20

26. A chemistry student is told to measure 12 grams of a milled substance for use during laboratory class. What would be appropriate to use?

(A) ruler
(B) scale
(C) beaker
(D) pipette

27. On a map, 1 inch = 120 miles. A traveler measures 4.3 inches as the distance between Hollywood, CA and Reno, NV. Estimate the driving distance in miles.

(A) 516
(B) 550
(C) 480
(D) 525

28. A student must attain a C grade average to pass. What is the independent variable in that sentence?

(A) pass
(B) average
(C) attain
(D) grade

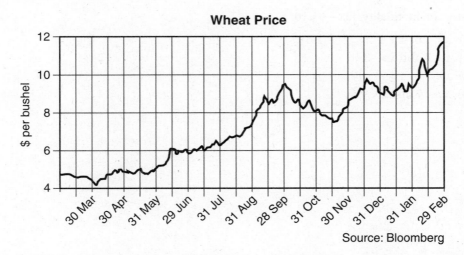

29. Based on the above graph, which date represents the last time the bushel of wheat was about $6?

(A) November 30
(B) July 31
(C) June 29
(D) May 31

30. Which graph would best display the average temperature changes throughout a year?

    (A) Gantt chart

    (B) line graph

    (C) pie chart

    (D) bar chart

31. Simplify the expression: $(3x^2 + 2x - 6) + (x^2 - 9x + 2)$.

    (A) $4x^2 - 7x - 4$

    (B) $2x^2 - 11x + 4$

    (C) $3x^2 + 11x + 8$

    (D) $x^2(2x - 3)$

32. Express the following into a mathematical expression: Sam is 7 years more than half his niece's age; if his niece's age is n, how old is Sam?

    (A) $\dfrac{n}{2} - 7 = x$

    (B) $2n + 7 = x$

    (C) $7\left(\dfrac{1}{2}n\right) = x$

    (D) $7 + \dfrac{n}{2} = x$

33. Solve this equation for y: $\dfrac{y}{3} = \dfrac{3}{9}$.

    (A) 1

    (B) 3

    (C) 6

    (D) 9

34. Solve the inequality: $|2x - 4| < 10$.

    (A) $x < 3$ or $x > 3$

    (B) $x < 7$ and $x > -3$

    (C) $x < 7$ or $x > 7$

    (D) $x > -7$ and $x < 7$

Part 3: Science

Time: 66 minutes

54 questions

QUESTIONS 1 AND 2 REFER TO THE PERIODIC TABLE.

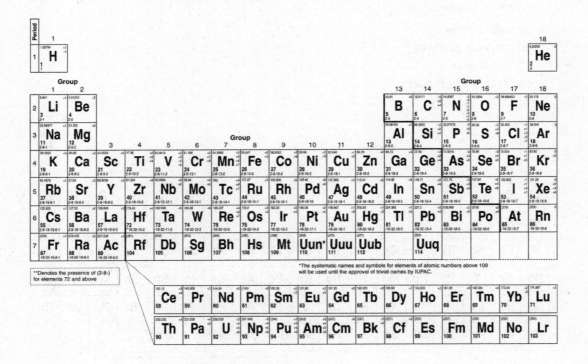

1. How many electrons does sodium (Na) have?

   (A) 4

   (B) 8

   (C) 11

   (D) 22

2. How many isotopes are possible with naturally occurring Zn? (Atomic weight is 65.38.)

   (A) 5

   (B) 12

   (C) 35

   (D) 50

3. What best explains the reason for ice caps forming on mountains and at the earth's poles?

(A) They both have arid climates.
(B) They both receive more of the sun's energy.
(C) The closeness to the sun increases snowfall.
(D) Mountains have a high elevation and ice caps receive indirect sunlight.

4. Which of these is the best example of potential energy that can be increased?

(A) rolling a bowling ball
(B) turning on a light bulb
(C) stretching a rubber band
(D) dropping a pencil

5. What is the model of enzyme action that describes the flexible fix of the enzyme-substrate complex?

(A) coenzymes
(B) enzyme pathway
(C) active site
(D) induced fit model

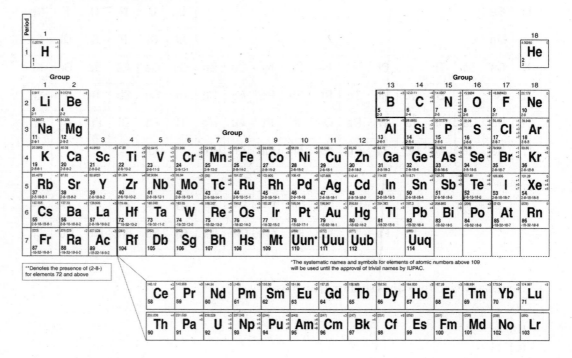

6. According to the above periodic table, if you move from left to right…

(A) atomic radii decrease
(B) atomic radii increase
(C) ionization energy decreases
(D) electronegativity decreases

7. The alkaline earth metals are located in the second row from the left and include elements such as Mg and Ca. Which of these are considered to be their specific chemical property?

(A) They want to keep an empty outer electron shell.
(B) They are most commonly found in the +1 oxidation state.
(C) They react with acids to release oxygen.
(D) They react with oxygen to form hydrogen peroxide.

8. A solution with a pH of 2 and testing red on litmus paper is considered to be

(A) a strong acid
(B) water
(C) a strong base
(D) a weak base

9. What is the name of a saturated hydrocarbon with 5 carbon atoms?

(A) methane
(B) propyne
(C) hexane
(D) pentane isopentane

10. Which is a common characteristic of the metalloids?

(A) may have metallic and nonmetallic properties
(B) bond slowly since the molecules are large
(C) always form covalent bonds
(D) are always saturated

11. When you balance this equation how many molecules of $CaCl_2$ will you have? ___$CaCL_2$ + ___Na_3PO_4 → ___$Ca_3(PO_4)_2$ + ___$NaCl$

(A) 2
(B) 3
(C) 4
(D) 6

12. What is specific heat?

(A) energy needed to raise water to 1°F
(B) the water standard for boiling point
(C) energy needed to raise any mass by 1°C
(D) heat required to vaporize a liquid

13. What is the degree of temperature called when a molecule change occurs from liquid to gas?

(A) centigrade
(B) freezing point
(C) latency
(D) kelvin

14. Of the research ideas listed below, which would be considered an hypothesis?

    (A) Noise levels distract students from effective study habits.
    (B) There is no relationship between maternal vitamin replacements and healthy outcomes for infants.
    (C) Taking medications as prescribed may be unnecessary for symptom management.
    (D) Hopefulness is worthlessness.

15. What type of research statement is this? "Increasing dietary HDL will decrease LDL in the blood of humans."

    (A) directional hypothesis
    (B) non-directional hypothesis
    (C) scientific argument
    (D) not a research question

16. What stage of the research process is this study? "Large caves were found in the area and the researchers suggest that any construction crew evaluate the possibility of a cave in. The area should be filled in before any major construction is attempted in the study area."

    (A) question asking
    (B) data collection
    (C) analysis
    (D) conclusion

17. Which research variable is the presumed cause?

    (A) independent
    (B) dependent
    (C) both independent and dependent
    (D) neither independent nor dependent

18. In a study called "What is the effect of diet on cancer?" what is the dependent variable?

    (A) diet
    (B) cancer
    (C) effect
    (D) both diet and cancer

19. There are stringent controls on this study of medication effects on high blood pressure. The data being collected is empirically based and very exact, with the study participants screened for factors that could be extraneous in nature. What type of study design is this?

    (A) either qualitative or quantitative
    (B) quantitative
    (C) qualitative
    (D) mixed design

20. A researcher is exploring the theory on chemical changes in heat between solids and gases. This study is based on scientific theory. What type of reasoning is this?

(A) quantitative
(B) deductive
(C) inductive
(D) proactive

21. The research team is considering a randomly assigned control group in the study. Which of these designs would fit?

(A) non-experimental design
(B) qualitative design
(C) experimental design
(D) survey

22. The researchers are attempting to formulate a scientific model or theory based on qualitative data. What would give the highest confidence in a theoretical model?

(A) There is transferability.
(B) The model fails the test in one area of the intervention.
(C) There is a researcher bias.
(D) The instrument is accurate and reflects the model's assumptions.

23. A person is watching the activities outside a department store. The researcher is recording behaviors of the customers. What type of study is this?

(A) quantitative
(B) qualitative
(C) descriptive
(D) experimental

24. Which classification in the biological classification system is always capitalized?

(A) family
(B) species
(C) kingdom
(D) genus

25. Why do organisms constantly adapt?

(A) so they can remove competition for food
(B) so they can reproduce without limits
(C) so they can get rid of predators
(D) so they can be better able to survive

26. Which of these cellular structures is not in the eukaryotic cell nucleus?

(A) chromatin
(B) nucleolus
(C) ribosomes
(D) nuclear membrane

27. Which cellular organelle controls what enters and leaves the cell?

    (A) mitochondrion
    (B) Golgi apparatus
    (C) nucleus
    (D) cell membrane

28. What is the picture of an individual's chromosomes called?

    (A) karyotype
    (B) chromatin
    (C) fingerprint
    (D) gene chart

29. During what phase of mitosis do the centromeres line up in the center of the cell for division to begin?

    (A) prophase
    (B) metaphase
    (C) anaphase
    (D) telophase

30. What is the jellylike interior of a cell called?

    (A) vacuole
    (B) cytoplasm
    (C) cytoskeleton
    (D) nucleus

31. What is a phenotype?

    (A) genetic code
    (B) physical appearance
    (C) ratio
    (D) parents

32. What type of parasitic relationship would not cause harm to the host?

    (A) mutualism
    (B) symbiosis
    (C) commensalism
    (D) pathogenicity

33. Which immunity is passed to the fetus inside the womb?

    (A) active acquired
    (B) passive acquired
    (C) innate
    (D) cell-mediated

34. A person has a blockage in the pulmonary artery. Which structure would blood back up into?

    (A) aorta
    (B) left ventricle
    (C) pulmonary veins
    (D) right ventricle

35. If a person had damage to the primary pacemaker cells of the heart, which area was damaged?

    (A) AV node
    (B) SA node
    (C) bundle of His
    (D) ventricles

36. What are the anchors of the atrioventricular valves of the heart?

    (A) chordae tendinae
    (B) great vessels
    (C) coronary ostia
    (D) trabeculae

37. What is the function of the ciliated mucosal membranes of the nasopharynx?

    (A) absorb air
    (B) humidify air
    (C) cool air
    (D) exchange gases

38. What is the movement of blood into and out of the capillary beds of the lungs to the body organs and tissues called?

    (A) perfusion
    (B) ventilation
    (C) diffusion
    (D) active transport

39. What is the maximum amount of gas that can be expired from the lung?

    (A) vital capacity
    (B) total lung capacity
    (C) functional capacity
    (D) residual volume

40. A twelve-year-old female notices her hair and skin feel more oily than normal. What hormone is responsible for the change in her sebaceous glands?

    (A) testosterone
    (B) estrogen
    (C) vitamin D
    (D) progesterone

41. What is *Tinea corporis* (ringworm)?

    (A) nematode infestation
    (B) fungal infection
    (C) viral infection
    (D) bacterial infection

42. Where are the glomeruli located within the kidney anatomical structure?

    (A) medulla
    (B) cortex
    (C) pyramids
    (D) columns

43. Why are proteins not usually present in urine?

    (A) All proteins filtered are subsequently reabsorbed.
    (B) All of the plasma proteins are too large to fit through the filtration slits.
    (C) All proteins filtered are subsequently degraded before elimination.
    (D) The negative charge of the glomerular filtration membrane repels the plasma proteins.

44. What is the trigone?

    (A) the orifice of the ureter
    (B) the inner area of the kidney
    (C) the triangular area between the openings of the two ureters and the urethra
    (D) the three divisions of the loop of Henle

45. Where does the axon leave the nerve cell body?

    (A) axon hillock
    (B) Nissl body
    (C) node of Ranvier
    (D) synaptic hillock

46. Which of the following transmit a nerve impulse at the highest rate?

    (A) large nonmyelinated axons
    (B) large myelinated axons
    (C) small nonmyelinated axons
    (D) small myelinated axons

47. Blocking which of the following neurotransmitters will reduce pain?

    (A) enkephalin
    (B) dopamine
    (C) acetylcholine
    (D) substance P

48. Where are the centers for maintenance of homeostasis and instinctive behavioral control located?

(A) thalamus
(B) medulla
(C) cerebellum
(D) hypothalamus

49. What force moves food down the esophagus?

(A) peristalsis
(B) retropulsion
(C) haustral segmentation
(D) defecation

50. Which sphincter keeps stomach acid from regurgitating into the esophagus?

(A) pyloric
(B) lower esophageal
(C) upper esophageal
(D) gastric

51. What changes occur in the aging gastrointestinal tract?

(A) decreased gastric juice secretion
(B) decreased gallbladder function
(C) increased liver size
(D) increased pancreas size

52. Antidiuretic hormone is important for what?

(A) the body's water balance and urine concentration
(B) maintaining electrolyte levels and concentrations
(C) follicular maturation
(D) regulation of metabolic processes

53. Where are target cells for oxytocin located?

(A) renal tubules
(B) thymus
(C) liver
(D) uterus

54. After birth, where are red blood cells normally made?

(A) liver and bone marrow
(B) liver and spleen
(C) bone marrow
(D) spleen and bone marrow

Part 4: English and Language Usage

■■■■■■■■■■■■■■■■■■■■■■■■■

Time: 34 minutes

34 questions

1. Abe _____ contacted Beth in their faraway home.

   Which of the following options correctly completes the sentence above?

   (A) lovingly
   (B) loving
   (C) lonesome
   (D) longing

2. <u>Connie</u> attended the casual gathering, but <u>her</u> new shoes seemed too classy.

   Which of the following correctly identifies the parts of speech in the underlined portions of the sentence above?

   (A) subject; clause
   (B) noun; pronoun
   (C) adjective; adverb
   (D) noun; object

3. Which of the following sentences has correct subject–verb agreement?

   (A) When arriving at the restaurant, he find the restroom first.
   (B) The reunion seldom linger, the family then retreats for the day.
   (C) When I yearningly want silence, the neighbor only gives me mayhem.
   (D) The club seems impartial at first but it only promote acquaintances.

4. Which of the following sentences provides an example of correct subject–verb agreement?

   (A) The faculty, upon analyzing applicant records, accept only the top 100.
   (B) The crowd, pleased with the show, cheer until the band comes back.
   (C) The team of participants are performing in orchestrated harmony.
   (D) The group of cyclists, viewing the intricate map, chooses the alternate trail.

5. When <u>Sam and Sally</u> finally met, ___ soon forgot all about the tiring long road. Which of the following options is the correct pronoun for the sentence above? The antecedent of the pronoun to be added is underlined.

   (A) them
   (B) he
   (C) she
   (D) they

6. While strolling with lovely Spin and Spot, Donna was stopped often by neighbors desiring to pet ___ dogs.

   Which of the following is the correct pronoun to complete the sentence above?

   (A) its
   (B) hers
   (C) her
   (D) them

7. Which of the following is an example of a correctly punctuated direct dialogue sentence?

   (A) Lana asked me "how long have you been waiting for me?"
   (B) Lana asked me, "How long have you been waiting for me?"
   (C) She asked me "How long have you been waiting for me"?
   (D) She asked me, how long have you been waiting for me?

8. Which of the following sentences correctly punctuates direct dialogue?

   (A) Sandy confided, "I'd rather read mystery over any other literary style."
   (B) I'd rather read mystery, confided Sandy, over any other literary style.
   (C) Sandy confided that "she'd rather read mystery" over any "other literary style."
   (D) "Over any other 'literary style,' I'd rather 'read mystery,'" confided Sandy.

9. Which of the following is an example of first-person point of view?

   (A) To avoid the heavy traffic, they decided to leave the concert toward the start of the last song.
   (B) To avoid the heavy traffic, Emmy and I decided to leave the concert when the last song started.
   (C) To avoid the heavy traffic, the couple decided to leave the concert as soon as the last song started.
   (D) You have to decide to leave the concert at the start of the last song to avoid the heavy traffic.

10. Which of the sentences in the instructions below is an example of third-person voice?

   (A) As soon as you see the curve, make a right and then a quick left turn.
   (B) Once anyone sees the curve, it is easy to make the right and quick left turns.
   (C) As soon as I missed the curve, there was no way to turn right and then left.
   (D) After we saw the curve, we failed to see the way to turn right and then left.

11. Chuck and Donna planned to retire. They bought some land. He found a well-paid job. She became an entrepreneur.

Which of the following options best uses grammar for style and clarity to combine the sentences above?

(A) Chuck and Donna planned to retire when they bought some land, yet he found a well-paid job, and she became an entrepreneur.

(B) Since Chuck and Donna planned to retire, they bought some land; nonetheless, he found a well-paid job and she became an entrepreneur.

(C) They bought some land when Chuck and Donna planned to retire; he found a well-paid job when she became an entrepreneur.

(D) They bought some land while they planned to retire; Donna became an entrepreneur while Chuck found a well-paid job.

12. They reached the springs. The waters were crystal clear. The day was dusking. They plunged in.

Which of the following options best uses grammar for style and clarity to combine the sentences above?

(A) When they reached the springs, the day was dusking; however, since the waters were crystal clear, they plunged in.

(B) They reached the springs, the waters were crystal clear and the day was dusking, so they plunged in.

(C) The day was dusking when they reached the springs, but they plunged in because the waters were crystal clear.

(D) When they reached the springs, the waters were crystal clear; though the day was dusking, they plunged in.

13. The variance was obvious, the team was green and the trainer was hoary.

Which of the following is the meaning of the word *hoary* as used in the sentence above?

(A) genial and strong
(B) gray or old
(C) casual and friendly
(D) corrupt or venal

14. In spite of all reviews, the results were immutable.

Which of the following is the meaning of the word *immutable*?

(A) unclear
(B) unsettled
(C) undecided
(D) unchangeable

15. After examining her aching leg, the examiner told her that it was related to osteitis.

In the sentence above, the prefix *oste-* indicates that the injury was related to what type of condition?

(A) bone irritation
(B) foot pain
(C) child ailment
(D) internal organ

16. The students were told that the condition of the patient was amnesia.

In the sentence above, the suffix *–ia* can best be defined by which of the following words?

(A) study of
(B) belief in
(C) state or condition
(D) a part of

17. Which of the following words is spelled correctly?

(A) axcessable
(B) endeering
(C) beleivable
(D) retrievable

18. Which of the following words is spelled correctly?

(A) benneficent
(B) malficent
(C) autonomous
(D) deduccion

19. He seemed _____ at first, but eventide markedly eased his reticence.

Which of the following options correctly completes the sentence above?

(A) prattling
(B) garrulous
(C) talkative
(D) taciturn

20. If they'd been _____, we'd be in the next town _____.

Which of the following options correctly completes the question above?

(A) altogether; all togethere
(B) all together; altogether
(C) all together; altogather
(D) altogether; all togetheir

21. And he offered burnt offering on the <u>alter</u>.

    Which of the following words corrects the spelling of the underlined word above?

    (A) alther
    (B) alto
    (C) altar
    (D) alder

22. Which of the following underlined words is an example of correct spelling?

    (A) Because her hair took longer in <u>dying</u>, her beautician kept her longer.
    (B) Her unconventional <u>genera</u> of novel writing was puzzling.
    (C) Because of the <u>stationary</u> nature of the road, he arrived late to the meeting.
    (D) Unlike your usual tardiness, <u>your</u> here early today.

23. Which of the following sentences follows the rules of capitalization?

    (A) I like the month of june.
    (B) I am with uncle Pete.
    (C) I am from the old South.
    (D) I'll be back in spring.

24. When we visit Germany, we'd like to enjoy the striking beauty of Heidelberg old City and an ancient structure, such as the ultimate fairytale castle landscape of Neuschwanstein.

    Which of the following words from the sentence above should be capitalized?

    (A) beauty
    (B) old
    (C) fairytale
    (D) castle

25. Which of the following sentences correctly applies the rules of punctuation?

    (A) I couldn't be on time, I overslept, the traffic was bad, the garage was full and I missed the train.
    (B) I couldn't be on time: I overslept, the traffic was bad, the garage was full, and I missed the train.
    (C) I couldn't be on time, I overslept; the traffic was bad, the garage was full, and I missed the train.
    (D) I couldn't be on time. I overslept, the traffic was bad, the garage was full; and I missed the train.

26. Your phone call was interrupted close to the phrase, "listen to me carefully, here's the address__"

    Which of the following punctuation marks correctly completes the sentence above?

    (A) ...
    (B) ,
    (C) .
    (D) :

27. Which of the following is an example of a simple sentence?

(A) The woman at the store.
(B) Questioned every price.
(C) The woman at the store who probed every price, berated everyone, and left first.
(D) The woman at the store probed every price, irked everyone, and left first.

28. Which of the following is an example of a simple sentence?

(A) The dog of the fluffy waggling tail had barked at the passerby joggers for the last half-hour, but he quieted down when I gave him a few crunchy treats.
(B) The dog of the fluffy waggling tail had barked at the passerby joggers for the last half-hour but quieted down with a few crunchy treats.
(C) The dog of fluffy waggling tail had barked at the passerby joggers for the last half-hour until I gave him a few crunchy treats.
(D) The dog of the fluffy waggling tail had barked at the passerby joggers for the last half-hour, though I gave him a few crunchy treats.

29. The visitors watched the fireworks. They were fascinated by the glittering display. Which of the following uses a conjunction to combine the sentences above so that the focus is more on the visitors' fascination and less on their watching the fireworks?

(A) The visitors watched the fireworks; they were fascinated by the glittering display.
(B) The visitors watched the fireworks and were fascinated by the glittering display.
(C) When the visitors watched the fireworks, they were fascinated by the glittering display.
(D) The visitors watched the fireworks, and they were fascinated by the glittering display.

30. The successful students in this program _____

Which of the following allows the above sentence to be completed as a simple sentence?

(A) do all their course assignments and seldom fall behind.
(B) do all their course assignments, and seldom fall behind.
(C) require no extra help, but ask detailed questions.
(D) require no extra help when their questions are satisfied.

31. Which of the following sentences is most clear and correct?

(A) In the nick of time the last cyclist arrived at the summit.
(B) The last cyclist reached the summit in the nick of time.
(C) The last cyclist reached the summit just in time.
(D) At the exact time, the last cyclist reached the summit.

32. We went to the new diner. Sitting was limited. The wait was long. We had a home meal.

    To improve sentence fluency, which of the following best states the information above in a single sentence?

    (A) We went to the new diner, sitting was limited and the wait was long, so we had a home meal.
    (B) When we went to the new diner and sitting was limited, the wait was long, then we had a home meal.
    (C) When sitting was limited and the wait was long, we had a home meal when we went to the new diner.
    (D) We went to the new diner and sitting was limited, since the wait was long we had a home meal.

33. I was discontented. I resigned my job. I went job hunting. I met interesting people.

    To improve sentence fluency, which of the following best states the information above in a single sentence?

    (A) I was discontented and resigned my job, so I went job hunting and met interesting people.
    (B) I was discontented, thus I resigned my job, so I went job hunting, and I met interesting people.
    (C) I went job hunting and I met interesting people when I was discontented, and I resigned my job.
    (D) I met interesting people when I went job hunting; as I was discontented, I resigned my job.

34. They drove to the lake. The journey was long. They slept on the way. They arrived early next day.

    To improve sentence fluency, which of the following best states the information above in a single sentence?

    (A) They drove to the lake, and the journey was long, they slept on the way, so they arrived early next day.
    (B) They drove to the lake and the journey was long, they arrived early next day because they slept on the way.
    (C) When they drove to the lake the journey was long, and they arrived early next day as they slept on the way.
    (D) The journey was long when they drove to the lake and, because they slept on the way, they arrived early next day.

ANSWER KEY
Practice Test 3

READING

1.	C	13.	B	25.	C	37.	B
2.	B	14.	B	26.	C	38.	A
3.	C	15.	B	27.	B	39.	C
4.	C	16.	C	28.	B	40.	B
5.	B	17.	D	29.	A	41.	A
6.	C	18.	A	30.	B	42.	D
7.	D	19.	B	31.	B	43.	A
8.	A	20.	B	32.	D	44.	C
9.	D	21.	C	33.	C	45.	A
10.	D	22.	D	34.	B	46.	B
11.	B	23.	A	35.	C	47.	D
12.	B	24.	B	36.	B	48.	D

MATHEMATICS

1.	D	10.	D	19.	C	28.	C
2.	A	11.	B	20.	B	29.	B
3.	B	12.	B	21.	A	30.	D
4.	B	13.	A	22.	D	31.	A
5.	A	14.	C	23.	C	32.	D
6.	C	15.	B	24.	B	33.	A
7.	D	16.	A	25.	D	34.	B
8.	B	17.	D	26.	B		
9.	A	18.	C	27.	A		

SCIENCE

1.	C	15.	A	29.	B	43.	B
2.	A	16.	D	30.	B	44.	C
3.	D	17.	A	31.	B	45.	A
4.	C	18.	B	32.	B	46.	B
5.	A	19.	B	33.	B	47.	D
6.	A	20.	B	34.	D	48.	B
7.	A	21.	C	35.	B	49.	A
8.	A	22.	A	36.	A	50.	B
9.	D	23.	C	37.	B	51.	B
10.	A	24.	D	38.	A	52.	A
11.	B	25.	D	39.	A	53.	D
12.	C	26.	C	40.	A	54.	C
13.	D	27.	D	41.	B		
14.	B	28.	A	42.	A		

ENGLISH AND LANGUAGE USAGE

1.	A	10.	B	19.	D	28.	B
2.	B	11.	A	20.	B	29.	C
3.	C	12.	C	21.	C	30.	A
4.	D	13.	B	22.	C	31.	B
5.	D	14.	D	23.	D	32.	D
6.	C	15.	A	24.	B	33.	A
7.	B	16.	C	25.	B	34.	B
8.	A	17.	D	26.	A		
9.	B	18.	C	27.	C		

ANSWER EXPLANATIONS
Reading

1. **(C)** The title represents a detail of the passage related to time of communications and change in the workplace. The theme was about the other person's ability to drive the daily activities of the workplace without being the official leader of the work unit.

2. **(B)** Narrative style tells a story. Expository passages explain a topic or subject in order to increase understanding of ideas. Technical writing usually addresses precise information. Persuasive writing tries to convince the reader to agree with the author.

3. **(C)** This is the general idea expressed by the author. The other choices reflect more incorrect assumptions not expressed in the passage.

4. **(C)** The author was trying to give an example of an inappropriate communication style. The other responses are contrary to the overall bias of the author.

5. **(B)** The passage describes events with a cause and effect structure. When one thing happens then another is likely to occur. The other statements describe facts or make general statements that are not directional.

6. **(C)** This response best describes the character's misinformation. The other responses reflect positive statements. Answer D was not mentioned in this passage.

7. **(D)** Persuasive writing tries to convince the reader to agree with the author. Expository passages explain a topic or subject in order to increase understanding of ideas. Technical writing usually addresses precise information. Narrative style tells a story.

8. **(A)** This was probably located in the introduction of this textbook since it appears to be an overview of the topic.

9. **(D)** If on a website, this would be found on an organizational site dealing with critical thinking. It is not associated with current events, government issues, or history of thinking.

10. **(D)** The only phrase that describes the topic is: "An organized way of thinking must be developed to direct our lives into clarity and direction." Answer A is a supporting argument, B is an opinion, and C is a question to capture the reader's attention.

11. **(B)** This is a supporting detail expressed by the author. The statement is too specific to be an overall topic, main idea, or theme.

12. **(B)** Universal usually focuses on consistency. With this writing sample it denotes consistency of interactions.

13. **(B)** The intended audience for this passage is cable subscribers.

14. **(B)** The false assumption is that tighter abdominal muscles mean weight loss, thus trying to convince the reader to purchase the item.

15. **(B)** This article discusses how to 'fool' the government where social security benefits are concerned.

16. **(C)** The reader should learn from the passage that some auto services can be done by the owner.

17. **(D)** The author is presenting an emotion in this passage.

18. **(A)** This passage is from a textbook since it is merely describing a fact.

19. **(B)** This passage is written to entertain, so it is from a novel. Since the unknown is explored it would be science fiction. It is not likely from a textbook since it is not purely informative in nature.

20. **(B)** The e-mail is written to offer a discount in price.

21. **(C)** The author's bias is that bundling is best.

22. **(D)** The definition in this context is to emphasize, rather than to pronounce the word with emphasis or to be fearful.

23. **(A)** Police Hall of Fame

24. **(B)** 112 minus 87 = 25 pages

25. **(C)** The national organization is being surveyed, as stated in the passage.

26. **(C)** 1998 was the year silver's price most closely aligned with silver's value.

27. **(B)** The child received the usual four-year-old immunizations, plus one extra from the special group that the child had not already received. Varicella, DTaP, MMR, Polio, and Meningococcal

28. **(B)** "Elementary" is between "electrical" and "engraving."

29. **(A)** The symbol for the AED is between these department stores.

30. **(B)** The only value that is three times the per serving amount is the fiber at 8 grams.

31. **(B)** The dinner meal is mentioned as the most expensive entertainment option.

32. **(D)** *Virtuosity* in this sentence means exceptional skill.

33. **(C)** The people are the only resource listed; the other terms are ways or rules for attaining the outcome.

34. **(B)** June is one of the months with the lowest precipitation in this area.

35. **(C)** The scale weight is 3.5 pounds.

36. **(B)** The thermometer will be read from the lowest end to the height of the colored fluid.

37. **(B)** Boston College at 7.6%

38. **(A)** This statement is located in "Everyday Learning." The other sections deal directly with "During the Test" or "After the Test."

39. **(C)** Multiple choice tests are composed of a specific test item.

40. **(B)** The National Institute of Health provides evidence-based information about ailments. Any online search would not give unbiased information. The commercial sites would provide biased information.

41. **(A)** This is a compound word.

42. **(D)** This is to add emphasis to the word.

43. **(A)** Even though there is an emphasis point entered on this chart, the highest amount of trading is early morning.

44. **(C)** "Recycling center" could be found between "recreational vehicles" and "rental cars."

45. **(A)** Cheese increased $5.61 a pound, sirloin steak only $5.47.

46. **(B)** This is a newspaper article so its purpose is to inform the reader.

47. **(D)** This ad is describing a component of event management. The other terms are topic details that describe parts of the entire job.

48. **(D)** Animals of New Zealand would be out of place in this reference since they are outside of the fauna of Asia.

Mathematics

1. **(D)** Simplify the expression with the innermost parentheses first. Then do the rest.

$$(9-2)^2 - 7 = 7^2 - 7$$
$$= 49 - 7$$
$$= 42$$

2. **(A)** $\dfrac{9 \times 4}{6 \times 3} = \dfrac{36}{18} = 2$

3. **(B)**

$$\begin{array}{r} 0.45 \\ -1.25 \\ \hline -0.80 \end{array}$$

When subtracting whole numbers, numbers are arranged in columns with like place values in each column.

4. **(B)** This option is correct. Thus,

$$\begin{array}{r} 4{,}313 \\ -2{,}635 \\ \hline 1{,}680 \end{array} \, .$$

5. **(A)** This is the only option; thus,

$$\begin{array}{r} 1{,}525{,}250 \\ -754{,}025 \\ \hline 771{,}225 \end{array}$$

6. **(C)** Since each tablet is 130 mg and 65 mg is ordered, there are two sets of 65 in each 130. Therefore the patient should receive 65/130 or ½ tablet.

7. **(D)** $4\dfrac{2}{3} - 3 = \dfrac{14}{3} - \dfrac{9}{3} = \dfrac{5}{3}$

8. **(B)** $\dfrac{\frac{8}{3}}{\frac{6}{5}} = \dfrac{8}{3} \times \dfrac{5}{6} = \dfrac{4}{3} \times \dfrac{5}{3} = \dfrac{20}{9} = 2.2222\ldots$

Change the division sign to a multiplication sign and flip the second fraction. Reduce factors in numerator with factors in denominator. Then multiply numerators together and denominators together.

9. **(A)** Rewrite the given expression by moving the decimal point to the right in both the dividend and divisor. So, $\frac{34}{465} = 0.0731182796$ or 0.073.

10. **(D)** The decimal form 5.1962 is greater than the square root of 25 and less than the square root of 36. Since option A is too small, the only option left is D.

11. **(B)** $0.15 \times n = 15$

$$n = \frac{15}{0.15}$$

$$n = 100$$

12. **(B)** $\frac{25}{1,000} = \frac{1}{40}$ in its simplest form.

13. **(A)** Since the largest number in the thousandths position is 5, the number 0.665 is greater than the other numbers.

14. **(C)** Since this is an estimate, start by simplifying to an easier number and compare. So, 88000/4700 = 18.72. Now observe: options A and B are too high and option D is too low, so the only possible option is C.

15. **(B)** (7453.21 + 2225.50 + 82.13 + 2.98) − (300 + 500 + 1500) = 9763.82 − 2300 = $7,463.82

16. **(A)** ($3,125.25 beginning salary) − (750 + 350.25 + 150.24 + 150.19 = $1,400.68 expenses) = $1,724.57 left from take-home salary

17. **(D)** Add all purchased items, thus

$10 ($5 × 2) + $3.50 + $1.50 + $6.50 + $2 = $23.50 .

18. **(C)** (50 × $4.40 = 220) + (50 × $6.50 = 325) + (20 × $7 = 140) = $685

19. **(C)** 654.19 × 0.073 = 47.75587 or $47.76

20. **(B)** If 35 students make up 100% of the class, then 5 students would make up 14.3% of the class.

21. **(A)** $\frac{160 \text{ miles}}{3 \text{ hours}} = \frac{D \text{ miles}}{7 \text{ hours}}$. Solving by cross-multiplying:

$$3 \times D = 160 \times 7 = \frac{3D}{3} = \frac{1,120}{3}$$

$D = 373.3$ miles.

22. **(D)** D = 500, C = 100, L = 50, X = 10, V = 5, I = 1. Traditionally, the numbers that follow in decreasing number add to the total number. Thus, DC = 600, LXXX = 80, IV = 4.

23. **(C)** M = 1,000, C = 100, X = 10, V = 5, I = 1. If a smaller number is listed before M, L, X, or V, it will be subtracted from the main number. Traditionally, the numbers that follow in decreasing number add to the total number. Thus, MM = 2,000, X = 10, IV = 4.

24. **(B)** 1 centimeter = 0.394 inches. Thus, 257 × 0.394 = 101.2 inches.

25. **(D)** 1 quart = 4 cups. So, 5 quarts = 20 cups.

26. **(B)** Since grams are weight measurements, scales would be appropriate in this case as these are used to measure weights of varied amounts.

27. **(A)** (4.3 inches × 120 miles)/1 inch = 516 miles

28. **(C)** The independent variable is the input that goes in the set of data.

29. **(B)** The last time the bushel of wheat was $6 was around July 31.

30. **(D)** A bar graph provides a way to compare higher/lower or a change in data over time.

31. **(A)** $(3x^2 + 2x - 6) + (x^2 - 9x + 2) = 3x^2 + x^2 + 2x - 9x - 6 + 2$

$$= 4x^2 - 7x - 4$$

32. **(D)** If Sam's niece is n years old, and he is 7 years older than half her age, Sam's age is $7 + \dfrac{n}{2}$.

33. **(A)** $\dfrac{y}{3} = \dfrac{3}{9}$

$$3\left(\dfrac{y}{3}\right) = 3\left(\dfrac{3}{9}\right)$$

$$y = 1$$

34. **(B)** $|2x - 4| < 10$

$2x - 4 + 10 < 10 + 4$

$2x > -6$ and $2x < 14$

$x > -3$ and $x < 7$

Since there is a greater than connector, the connecting word is *and*, not *or*.

Science

1. **(C)** Sodium has eleven electrons according to the periodic chart.

2. **(A)** The atomic weight of Zn is 65; its atomic number is 30. 30–35 neutrons means five possible isotopes.

3. **(D)** The heat of the sun is received on the mountaintops but the higher the elevation, the colder the temperatures. The polar ice caps exist because they receive solar energy indirectly.

4. **(C)** The rubber band when released has an increased potential energy. The other objects have a static amount of energy.

5. **(A)** The induced fit model is an explanation of why a flexible substrate allows for the enzyme-substrate complex.

6. **(A)** If you move from left to right on the periodic table, atomic radii decrease.

7. **(A)** The alkaline earth metals have two valence electrons, are willing to give them up to achieve an empty outer orbit, are more reactive as the list progresses downward, and react with acids to form salts and release hydrogen.

8. **(A)** pH values of less than 7 are considered to be acidic with smaller numbers proportionally increasing the strength of an acid. pH of 2 is a strong acid. Litmus paper measures acid as red and a base as blue.

9. **(D)** Saturated hydrocarbons end in -*ane* with the number of carbon atoms delineated in the prefix of the chemical's name. (*eth* = 2, *but* = 4, *pent* = 5, *hex* = 6)

10. **(A)** Metalloids have metallic and nonmetallic properties and bond readily.

11. **(B)** Start with the calcium and you will find that there are three on the other side of the equation. Then cross-check the other side for totals of Ca and Cl.

12. **(C)** Specific heat is the energy needed to raise any mass by 1°C. Water has the second highest specific heat.

13. **(D)** Degrees kelvin is the temperature at the conversion in Centigrade plus 273.

14. **(B)** Hypotheses usually make predictions and are well defined.

15. **(A)** This statement sets the direction for the research, makes a prediction, and is well defined.

16. **(D)** These researchers have already concluded that the area being explored is dangerous and are making recommendations based on their data analysis.

17. **(A)** The independent variable is the change agent.

 18. **(B)** The dependent variable is cancer. It is dependent on you doing something independent to stop the process.

19. **(B)** The empirical detail and control of this study make it quantitative in nature.

20. **(B)** When you start research based on an existing theory, it is called deductive reasoning.

21. **(C)** This is an experimental design technique commonly used in intervention studies to make sure the effect was without researcher bias.

22. **(A)** Qualitative studies are considered to be reliable if the data can be applied to many groups.

23. **(C)** The study is descriptive.

24. **(D)** The genus classification in the biological classification system is always capitalized.

25. **(D)** Adaptation is a necessity for survival.

26. **(C)** Ribosomes are located within the cell and are not surrounded by the nuclear membrane.

27. **(D)** The cellular membrane controls what enters and leaves the cell. The vesicles are the transport mechanisms.

28. **(A)** The picture of an individual's chromosomes is called a karyotype.

29. **(B)** During metaphase, the centromeres line up in the center of the cell for division to begin.

30. **(B)** Cytoplasm is the jellylike interior of a cell.

31. **(B)** The phenotype is the physical expression of the genetic traits.

32. **(B)** A pathogen that is not harmful to the host is symbiotic.

33. **(B)** Passive immunity is passed without introducing the substance directly into the organism.

34. **(D)** The pulmonary artery provided blood from the right side of the heart to be oxygenated.

35. **(B)** The SA (sinoatrial) node is the pacemaker of the heart.

36. **(A)** The chordae tendinea secure the atrioventricular valves of the heart to the heart wall.

37. **(B)** The function of the ciliated mucosal membranes of the nasopharynx is to humidify air.

38. **(A)** The movement of blood into and out of the capillary beds of the lungs to the body organs and tissues is called perfusion.

39. **(A)** Vital capacity is the maximum amount of gas that can be expired from the lung.

40. **(A)** Testosterone is the hormone responsible for changes in her sebaceous glands at puberty.

41. **(B)** *Tinea corporis* (ringworm) is a fungal infection.

42. **(A)** The glomeruli are located within the kidney medulla.

43. **(B)** Proteins are not usually present in urine because all of the plasma proteins are too large to fit through the filtration slits.

44. **(C)** The trigone is a triangular area between the openings of the two ureters and the urethra.

45. **(A)** The axon leaves the nerve cell body at the axon hillock.

46. **(B)** Large myelinated axons transmit a nerve impulse at the highest rate.

47. **(D)** Substance P will block pain.

48. **(B)** The medulla maintains homeostasis and controls instinctive behavior.

49. **(A)** Peristalsis moves food down the esophagus.

50. **(B)** The lower esophageal sphincter keeps stomach acid from regurgitating into the esophagus.

51. **(B)** Decreased gallbladder function occurs in the aging gastrointestinal tract.

52. **(A)** Antidiuretic hormone is important in the body's water balance and urine concentration.

53. **(D)** The target cells for oxytocin are located in the uterus. The hormone stimulates uterine contractions after birth.

54. **(C)** After birth, red blood cells are normally made only in the bone marrow.

English and Language Usage

1. **(A)** This option contains the proper adjective *lovingly* to complete the sentence. The other options are incorrect in either grammar or case.

2. **(B)** This option correctly identifies *Connie* as a noun and *her* as a pronoun.

3. **(C)** This option contains correct subject–verb agreement: "I… want" and "the neighbor… gives." All other options contain incorrect subject–verb agreement with regard to number or case.

4. **(D)** This option contains correct subject–verb agreement: "the group… chooses." All other options contain incorrect subject–verb agreement with regard to number.

5. **(D)** The antecedent, *Sam and Sally*, is plural and neutral, which means that *they* is the only correct answer. All other options are incorrect in terms of number, gender, or case.

6. **(C)** This option correctly completes the sentence as it contains the correct pronoun to use. All other options are incorrect pronouns to use in this case.

7. **(B)** This option correctly contains double quotation marks around the whole quote. Option A does not introduce the quotation with a comma, and option C contains quotations in the wrong places. Option D has no quotation marks to properly indicate direct dialogue.

8. **(A)** This option correctly contains double quotation marks around the whole quote. Option B has no quotation marks to properly indicate direct dialogue, option C contains quotations in the wrong places, and option D unnecessarily adds single quotes.

9. **(B)** This option is an example of first-person point of view. Options A and C are examples of third-person point of view. Option D is an example of second-person point of view.

10. **(B)** This option is an example of third-person point of view. Option A is an example of second-person point of view. Options C and D are examples of first-person point of view.

11. **(A)** This option effectively uses transitional words to combine the sentences into a single sentence to reflect the original meaning of the group of sentences. All other options may lead to confusion of the writer's original intent.

12. **(C)** This option effectively uses transitional words to combine the sentences into a single sentence that still reflects the original meaning of the group of sentences.

13. **(B)** This option rightly and properly defines the word *hoary* (which has nothing to do with venal or unscrupulous behavior). All other options are incorrect.

14. **(D)** This option correctly defines the word *immutable*. All other options are incorrect.

15. **(A)** The prefix *oste-* (or *osteo-*) originates from the Greek language. The word *osteitis* means "inflammation of bone." Therefore, it can be concluded that this person had symptoms of bone irritation.

16. **(C)** The suffix *-ia* originates from the Latin language. The word *amnesia* means "state or condition of forgetfulness." Therefore, it can be concluded that this patient was not necessarily good at recalling.

17. **(D)** This option is the correct spelling: *retrievable* is a commonly misspelled word: its root word (*retrieve*) ends in *e*, which must be dropped before adding *-able*.

18. **(C)** This option alone is spelled correctly.

19. **(D)** This option contains the correct word that completes the given sentence. The phrase "eased his reticence" adds strength to the meaning of *taciturn*.

20. **(B)** This option contains the only word set that completes the given sentence. *All together* and *altogether* are commonly misspelled and misused homophone (sound alike) words.

21. **(C)** This option is spelled correctly; *altar* is a commonly misspelled word. The preposition *on* ("atop, onto, over, upon") offers a cue to identify *altar* as the correctly spelled word.

22. **(C)** This option is spelled correctly. All other options are commonly misspelled words: *dying* ("about to die") is not *dyeing* ("coloring"); *genera* ("plural of *genus*") is not *genre* ("literary category"); and *your* (possessive pronoun) is not *you're* (contraction of *you are*).

23. **(D)** Because names of seasons are only capitalized when used in a title or personified in poetry, the word *spring* in this case is properly not capitalized. None of the other options follow correct rules of capitalization.

24. **(B)** The word *old* should be capitalized, as it is used as a proper noun in this context. There is no need to capitalize the words in options A, C, or D.

25. **(B)** This option is correctly punctuated with a colon heralding a list, and phrases in a series separated by a comma.

26. **(A)** To correctly punctuate the sentence, ellipses (…) are required. They are used to signal a trailing or unfinished thought, or to denote omission of words in a conversation within a quotation, as in this case.

27. **(C)** This option is constructed as a simple sentence containing one subject and one verb. Although the sentence is detailed, there are no clauses adding to the complexity of the sentence structure, as is the case in option D. Options A and B are not complete sentences.

28. **(B)** This option is constructed as a simple sentence with one subject and a compound verb. Although the sentence is detailed, there are no clauses adding to the complexity of the sentence structure, as in the case of all other options.

29. **(C)** This option makes one clause subordinate to the other by the addition of a subordinating conjunction. All other options contain two clauses of equal weight.

30. **(A)** This option completes the sentence as a simple sentence. All other options are examples of compound sentences.

31. **(B)** This option clearly and succinctly conveys the writer's intent to accurately describe the event. The other options are written in ways in which the writer's intent might be confused.

32. **(D)** This option is an example of the use of grammar to enhance clarity and readability. The four sentences are combined into one clear, succinct sentence that is easy to read and understand. The other options, while employing correct grammar to condense the four sentences, do not do so in a manner that clearly expresses the writer's intent.

33. **(A)** This option effectively uses transitional words to combine the sentences into a single sentence that still reflects the original meaning of the group of sentences.

34. **(B)** This option effectively uses transitional words to combine the sentences into a single sentence that still reflects the original meaning of the group of sentences.

ANSWER SHEET
Practice Test 4

READING

1. Ⓐ Ⓑ Ⓒ Ⓓ	13. Ⓐ Ⓑ Ⓒ Ⓓ	25. Ⓐ Ⓑ Ⓒ Ⓓ	37. Ⓐ Ⓑ Ⓒ Ⓓ
2. Ⓐ Ⓑ Ⓒ Ⓓ	14. Ⓐ Ⓑ Ⓒ Ⓓ	26. Ⓐ Ⓑ Ⓒ Ⓓ	38. Ⓐ Ⓑ Ⓒ Ⓓ
3. Ⓐ Ⓑ Ⓒ Ⓓ	15. Ⓐ Ⓑ Ⓒ Ⓓ	27. Ⓐ Ⓑ Ⓒ Ⓓ	39. Ⓐ Ⓑ Ⓒ Ⓓ
4. Ⓐ Ⓑ Ⓒ Ⓓ	16. Ⓐ Ⓑ Ⓒ Ⓓ	28. Ⓐ Ⓑ Ⓒ Ⓓ	40. Ⓐ Ⓑ Ⓒ Ⓓ
5. Ⓐ Ⓑ Ⓒ Ⓓ	17. Ⓐ Ⓑ Ⓒ Ⓓ	29. Ⓐ Ⓑ Ⓒ Ⓓ	41. Ⓐ Ⓑ Ⓒ Ⓓ
6. Ⓐ Ⓑ Ⓒ Ⓓ	18. Ⓐ Ⓑ Ⓒ Ⓓ	30. Ⓐ Ⓑ Ⓒ Ⓓ	42. Ⓐ Ⓑ Ⓒ Ⓓ
7. Ⓐ Ⓑ Ⓒ Ⓓ	19. Ⓐ Ⓑ Ⓒ Ⓓ	31. Ⓐ Ⓑ Ⓒ Ⓓ	43. Ⓐ Ⓑ Ⓒ Ⓓ
8. Ⓐ Ⓑ Ⓒ Ⓓ	20. Ⓐ Ⓑ Ⓒ Ⓓ	32. Ⓐ Ⓑ Ⓒ Ⓓ	44. Ⓐ Ⓑ Ⓒ Ⓓ
9. Ⓐ Ⓑ Ⓒ Ⓓ	21. Ⓐ Ⓑ Ⓒ Ⓓ	33. Ⓐ Ⓑ Ⓒ Ⓓ	45. Ⓐ Ⓑ Ⓒ Ⓓ
10. Ⓐ Ⓑ Ⓒ Ⓓ	22. Ⓐ Ⓑ Ⓒ Ⓓ	34. Ⓐ Ⓑ Ⓒ Ⓓ	46. Ⓐ Ⓑ Ⓒ Ⓓ
11. Ⓐ Ⓑ Ⓒ Ⓓ	23. Ⓐ Ⓑ Ⓒ Ⓓ	35. Ⓐ Ⓑ Ⓒ Ⓓ	47. Ⓐ Ⓑ Ⓒ Ⓓ
12. Ⓐ Ⓑ Ⓒ Ⓓ	24. Ⓐ Ⓑ Ⓒ Ⓓ	36. Ⓐ Ⓑ Ⓒ Ⓓ	48. Ⓐ Ⓑ Ⓒ Ⓓ

MATHEMATICS

1. Ⓐ Ⓑ Ⓒ Ⓓ	10. Ⓐ Ⓑ Ⓒ Ⓓ	19. Ⓐ Ⓑ Ⓒ Ⓓ	28. Ⓐ Ⓑ Ⓒ Ⓓ
2. Ⓐ Ⓑ Ⓒ Ⓓ	11. Ⓐ Ⓑ Ⓒ Ⓓ	20. Ⓐ Ⓑ Ⓒ Ⓓ	29. Ⓐ Ⓑ Ⓒ Ⓓ
3. Ⓐ Ⓑ Ⓒ Ⓓ	12. Ⓐ Ⓑ Ⓒ Ⓓ	21. Ⓐ Ⓑ Ⓒ Ⓓ	30. Ⓐ Ⓑ Ⓒ Ⓓ
4. Ⓐ Ⓑ Ⓒ Ⓓ	13. Ⓐ Ⓑ Ⓒ Ⓓ	22. Ⓐ Ⓑ Ⓒ Ⓓ	31. Ⓐ Ⓑ Ⓒ Ⓓ
5. Ⓐ Ⓑ Ⓒ Ⓓ	14. Ⓐ Ⓑ Ⓒ Ⓓ	23. Ⓐ Ⓑ Ⓒ Ⓓ	32. Ⓐ Ⓑ Ⓒ Ⓓ
6. Ⓐ Ⓑ Ⓒ Ⓓ	15. Ⓐ Ⓑ Ⓒ Ⓓ	24. Ⓐ Ⓑ Ⓒ Ⓓ	33. Ⓐ Ⓑ Ⓒ Ⓓ
7. Ⓐ Ⓑ Ⓒ Ⓓ	16. Ⓐ Ⓑ Ⓒ Ⓓ	25. Ⓐ Ⓑ Ⓒ Ⓓ	34. Ⓐ Ⓑ Ⓒ Ⓓ
8. Ⓐ Ⓑ Ⓒ Ⓓ	17. Ⓐ Ⓑ Ⓒ Ⓓ	26. Ⓐ Ⓑ Ⓒ Ⓓ	
9. Ⓐ Ⓑ Ⓒ Ⓓ	18. Ⓐ Ⓑ Ⓒ Ⓓ	27. Ⓐ Ⓑ Ⓒ Ⓓ	

SCIENCE

1. Ⓐ Ⓑ Ⓒ Ⓓ   15. Ⓐ Ⓑ Ⓒ Ⓓ   29. Ⓐ Ⓑ Ⓒ Ⓓ   43. Ⓐ Ⓑ Ⓒ Ⓓ
2. Ⓐ Ⓑ Ⓒ Ⓓ   16. Ⓐ Ⓑ Ⓒ Ⓓ   30. Ⓐ Ⓑ Ⓒ Ⓓ   44. Ⓐ Ⓑ Ⓒ Ⓓ
3. Ⓐ Ⓑ Ⓒ Ⓓ   17. Ⓐ Ⓑ Ⓒ Ⓓ   31. Ⓐ Ⓑ Ⓒ Ⓓ   45. Ⓐ Ⓑ Ⓒ Ⓓ
4. Ⓐ Ⓑ Ⓒ Ⓓ   18. Ⓐ Ⓑ Ⓒ Ⓓ   32. Ⓐ Ⓑ Ⓒ Ⓓ   46. Ⓐ Ⓑ Ⓒ Ⓓ
5. Ⓐ Ⓑ Ⓒ Ⓓ   19. Ⓐ Ⓑ Ⓒ Ⓓ   33. Ⓐ Ⓑ Ⓒ Ⓓ   47. Ⓐ Ⓑ Ⓒ Ⓓ
6. Ⓐ Ⓑ Ⓒ Ⓓ   20. Ⓐ Ⓑ Ⓒ Ⓓ   34. Ⓐ Ⓑ Ⓒ Ⓓ   48. Ⓐ Ⓑ Ⓒ Ⓓ
7. Ⓐ Ⓑ Ⓒ Ⓓ   21. Ⓐ Ⓑ Ⓒ Ⓓ   35. Ⓐ Ⓑ Ⓒ Ⓓ   49. Ⓐ Ⓑ Ⓒ Ⓓ
8. Ⓐ Ⓑ Ⓒ Ⓓ   22. Ⓐ Ⓑ Ⓒ Ⓓ   36. Ⓐ Ⓑ Ⓒ Ⓓ   50. Ⓐ Ⓑ Ⓒ Ⓓ
9. Ⓐ Ⓑ Ⓒ Ⓓ   23. Ⓐ Ⓑ Ⓒ Ⓓ   37. Ⓐ Ⓑ Ⓒ Ⓓ   51. Ⓐ Ⓑ Ⓒ Ⓓ
10. Ⓐ Ⓑ Ⓒ Ⓓ   24. Ⓐ Ⓑ Ⓒ Ⓓ   38. Ⓐ Ⓑ Ⓒ Ⓓ   52. Ⓐ Ⓑ Ⓒ Ⓓ
11. Ⓐ Ⓑ Ⓒ Ⓓ   25. Ⓐ Ⓑ Ⓒ Ⓓ   39. Ⓐ Ⓑ Ⓒ Ⓓ   53. Ⓐ Ⓑ Ⓒ Ⓓ
12. Ⓐ Ⓑ Ⓒ Ⓓ   26. Ⓐ Ⓑ Ⓒ Ⓓ   40. Ⓐ Ⓑ Ⓒ Ⓓ   54. Ⓐ Ⓑ Ⓒ Ⓓ
13. Ⓐ Ⓑ Ⓒ Ⓓ   27. Ⓐ Ⓑ Ⓒ Ⓓ   41. Ⓐ Ⓑ Ⓒ Ⓓ
14. Ⓐ Ⓑ Ⓒ Ⓓ   28. Ⓐ Ⓑ Ⓒ Ⓓ   42. Ⓐ Ⓑ Ⓒ Ⓓ

ENGLISH AND LANGUAGE USAGE

1. Ⓐ Ⓑ Ⓒ Ⓓ   10. Ⓐ Ⓑ Ⓒ Ⓓ   19. Ⓐ Ⓑ Ⓒ Ⓓ   28. Ⓐ Ⓑ Ⓒ Ⓓ
2. Ⓐ Ⓑ Ⓒ Ⓓ   11. Ⓐ Ⓑ Ⓒ Ⓓ   20. Ⓐ Ⓑ Ⓒ Ⓓ   29. Ⓐ Ⓑ Ⓒ Ⓓ
3. Ⓐ Ⓑ Ⓒ Ⓓ   12. Ⓐ Ⓑ Ⓒ Ⓓ   21. Ⓐ Ⓑ Ⓒ Ⓓ   30. Ⓐ Ⓑ Ⓒ Ⓓ
4. Ⓐ Ⓑ Ⓒ Ⓓ   13. Ⓐ Ⓑ Ⓒ Ⓓ   22. Ⓐ Ⓑ Ⓒ Ⓓ   31. Ⓐ Ⓑ Ⓒ Ⓓ
5. Ⓐ Ⓑ Ⓒ Ⓓ   14. Ⓐ Ⓑ Ⓒ Ⓓ   23. Ⓐ Ⓑ Ⓒ Ⓓ   32. Ⓐ Ⓑ Ⓒ Ⓓ
6. Ⓐ Ⓑ Ⓒ Ⓓ   15. Ⓐ Ⓑ Ⓒ Ⓓ   24. Ⓐ Ⓑ Ⓒ Ⓓ   33. Ⓐ Ⓑ Ⓒ Ⓓ
7. Ⓐ Ⓑ Ⓒ Ⓓ   16. Ⓐ Ⓑ Ⓒ Ⓓ   25. Ⓐ Ⓑ Ⓒ Ⓓ   34. Ⓐ Ⓑ Ⓒ Ⓓ
8. Ⓐ Ⓑ Ⓒ Ⓓ   17. Ⓐ Ⓑ Ⓒ Ⓓ   26. Ⓐ Ⓑ Ⓒ Ⓓ
9. Ⓐ Ⓑ Ⓒ Ⓓ   18. Ⓐ Ⓑ Ⓒ Ⓓ   27. Ⓐ Ⓑ Ⓒ Ⓓ

Part 1: Reading

Time: 58 minutes

48 questions

QUESTIONS 1 THROUGH 6 ARE BASED ON THE FOLLOWING PASSAGE.

Dreaming with a Purpose

There are many reasons for dreams. There are many theories that exist about dreams that are unproven. Some believe that dreams are important messages about ourselves or about situations that we have experienced.

Lucid dreams are ones that allow you to know that you are dreaming. Some people may control their own dreams through the process of dreaming about previous dreams or recreating a waking dream based on the topic of the dream. Critics believe that lucid dreams exist because someone ascribes to the existence of them. Research into the benefits of this technique established its use in nightmares or sleep paralysis.

There are programs available to help people control their dreams with waking dream logs and special sound emissions to encourage lucidity. For example, a person might dream of monsters and then with the lucid dream technique turn the monster into a wonderful person. The theory is that if dreams can be remembered, then they can also be re-experienced; therefore some of the anxiety associated with the dream may be diminished through re-enactment and a change in the situation or focus of the dream.

1. Which phrase from the above passage best represents the overall theme?

    (A) dreaming with a purpose
    (B) re-enactment and change
    (C) lucid dreams exist
    (D) messages and nightmares

2. The above passage demonstrates which writing type?

    (A) expository
    (B) narrative
    (C) persuasive
    (D) technical

3. What precise explanation is this passage presenting?

    (A) Lucid dreaming is not a reality.
    (B) Logs for remembering dreams are widely used.
    (C) Lucidity could be a dangerous undertaking.
    (D) Lucid dreams may be enlightening.

4. What is a bias expressed in the passage?

(A) We can turn monsters into wonderful people.
(B) All people can control their dreams.
(C) Lucid dreams exist because someone ascribes to the existence of them.
(D) Forgetting dreams are the only way to control dreams.

5. Which sentence from the above passage is most reflective of a description text structure?

(A) Some believe that dreams are important messages about ourselves or about situations that we have experienced.
(B) Critics believe that lucid dreams exist because someone ascribes to the existence of them.
(C) For example, a person might dream of monsters and then with the lucid dream technique turn the monster into a wonderful person.
(D) Lucid dreams are ones that allow you to know that you are dreaming.

6. Which of these statements is an example of the writer's logic about lucid dreaming?

(A) Dream control can be beneficial for everyone.
(B) Dream logs should be used.
(C) Lucid dreams are positive phenomena.
(D) Lucid dream control can help decrease anxiety for some.

QUESTIONS 7 THROUGH 11 ARE BASED ON THE FOLLOWING PASSAGE.

The Athlete

Jack was five feet tall and just the right weight to be a jockey. He was asked to train and decided in favor of the endeavor. He didn't expect to win any races but hoped to at least show. He secretly dreamed of at least one win. His surprise was overwhelming when he won a few races early in the season. There was a horse available for the Kentucky Derby so he begged for the opportunity.

After running at second place for the majority of the race, he inched forward and slumped in the saddle. The fans were surprised when it was discovered that Jack had a stroke before winning the race and was unconscious when crossing the finish line. The horse was the real winner. When later asked about the event and consequences, Jack told the press that it was great to win a race even if it isn't remembered as expected.

7. This news article would most likely be published in which section of the newspaper?

(A) news makers
(B) editorial
(C) world news reports
(D) football today

8. Why was this passage written?

(A) to introduce a subject
(B) to entertain
(C) to persuade
(D) to report facts

9. Identify a phrase that would be a primary source of information in this passage.

   (A) He secretly dreamed of at least one win.
   (B) When later asked about the event and consequences,
   (C) The horse was the real winner.
   (D) It was discovered that Jack had a stroke before winning the race.

10. Which can be identified as an author's bias in this passage?

    (A) Jack was five feet tall and just the right weight to be a jockey.
    (B) The horse was the real winner.
    (C) He secretly dreamed of at least one win.
    (D) He was asked to train and decided in favor of the endeavor.

11. "The horse was the real winner." Which term best describes this quote?

    (A) topic
    (B) supporting detail
    (C) main idea
    (D) theme

There is an organic line of face products that you can buy at the better department stores and online. I use this soap and moisturizing oil. I massage it on my skin in the morning and it's amazing. I also use the eye cream. I love the iridescent glow of the natural lipgloss on my eyelids. I guess I just love the organics and I'm really excited about the newest fruit scented deodorants!

12. According to the above passage, what is the author's overall conclusion about organic skin care products?

    (A) Disappointed that there are too few.
    (B) They are too expensive.
    (C) They must be used for their intended purpose only.
    (D) Excited about every product available.

Having trouble keeping up with your personal training and fitness? There are many electronic devices to help out. These devices come at a hefty price but can help the athlete or anyone wanting to track activity to improve performance. One device will monitor your ability to sit up straight and softly vibrate if you slouch. Another new device will let you track your ability to kick effectively or hit a tennis ball harder. Keep reading this journal to discover even more innovative approaches to fitness.

13. The above passage is most probably an example of an article from what type of published work?

    (A) health newsletter
    (B) internet add
    (C) travel magazine
    (D) medical journal

This modern wristband motivates you to achieve your fitness goals by calculating steps taken, calories burned, and distance traveled throughout the day. It lightens up to alert you and others as you progress. The device wirelessly syncs your stats to your computer or smart phone, then measures hours and quality of sleep before silently waking you in the morning.

14. What is the message implied in the above passage?

   (A) The reader needs to be awakened at a set time.
   (B) The reader wants to track progress.
   (C) Continuous monitoring is beneficial.
   (D) Others should be alerted when you succeed.

Don't work so hard in college that you lose track of the real goal. The real goal is to finish with a degree. Are you having problems achieving a 4.0 average? Many trade schools evaluate you on your ability to finish rather than your grade point average. Please do try to maintain at least a 3.0 average, but only try to get above that average if you are planning on attending a law or medical college.

15. The advising staff prepared the above in a presentation to high school students. What is the take away message?

   (A) Your grade point average is extremely important.
   (B) Don't work too hard in school.
   (C) Trade occupations expect a 4.0 grade point average.
   (D) A lower grade point average is needed for medical school.

We all drive or run too fast. Why not slow down and enjoy the world we live in? The breath of fresh air you inhale after a cool rain on a mountaintop can really change your perspective on life. The effects of the breeze on the leaves surrounding the trees in your local park can lift you beyond this meager existence into a spiritual experience. Ever listen to the crackle of the wood in a fireplace? Seek peace in your everyday and leave the speed behind.

16. Which answer describes the above passage's general message?

   (A) The reader should slow down and experience life.
   (B) The reader should take a vacation.
   (C) The reader should walk in the cool rain.
   (D) The reader should speed more and slow down less.

This quotation by John Gardner is an example of how a few words can mean so much: "Life is the art of drawing without an eraser." In it you can detect a passion for living without regrets and without the need to change anything from the past.

17. Why is the author using a quotation in the above text?

   (A) to entertain
   (B) to inform
   (C) to persuade
   (D) to express emotion

As she approached the scene of the crime there was a damp unique odor coming from the side of the car. Upon opening the door a soft cry was audible and a cat escaped from the scene. A sudden explosion shot her back into the driveway of the house next door.

18. Which type of literature is the above passage most likely from?

   (A) textbook
   (B) science fiction novel
   (C) research journal
   (D) mystery novel

We do know that bullying is a problem that reaches into the culture, community, school, peer groups, and families. The extent of the problem will vary across different communities and schools. We should remember that a famous Norwegian researcher who started studying bullying in the early 1980 s, did so partly as a result of three boys, ages 10 to 14, who committed suicide in 1982 as a result of being bullied. Sadly, this is not a new problem.

19. Which type of literature is the above passage most likely from?

   (A) textbook
   (B) science fiction novel
   (C) research journal
   (D) mystery novel

QUESTIONS 20 AND 21 ARE BASED ON THE FOLLOWING E-MAIL.

Customer,

We cannot grant you your bonus air miles since you have not subscribed to bonus miles on your charge account. Please enroll and pay your annual fee, and you will have these miles for future travels. We don't want you to be left behind at your next travel opportunity because of your inability to redeem the travel bonuses.

Enroll by visiting this site!

---

20. What is the main purpose of this e-mail?

   (A) The author wants to sell bonus miles.
   (B) The author wants to offer a discount in price.
   (C) The author disagrees with the way the customer enrolled.
   (D) The author wants the customer to sign up to receive the bonus.

21. What is the author's bias regarding the option mentioned in the e-mail?

   (A) It's best to accumulate bonus miles.
   (B) Bonus time is accrued without extra effort.
   (C) He thinks the customer should stay at home.
   (D) There are no biases noted.

Sift together flour, baking powder, and salt. Set aside. Place butter and sugar in large bowl of electric stand mixer and beat until light in color. Add egg and milk and beat to combine. Put mixer on low speed, gradually add flour, and beat until mixture pulls away from the side of the bowl. Divide the dough in half, wrap in waxed paper, and refrigerate for 2 hours.

Preheat oven to 375 degrees F.

Sprinkle surface where you will roll out dough with powdered sugar. Remove 1 wrapped pack of dough from refrigerator at a time, sprinkle rolling pin with powdered sugar, and roll out dough to 1/4-inch thick. Move the dough around and check underneath frequently to make sure it is not sticking. Cut into desired shape, place at least 1-inch apart on greased baking sheet, parchment, or silicone baking mat, and bake for 7 to 9 minutes or until cookies are just beginning to turn brown around the edges, rotating cookie sheet halfway through baking time. Let sit on baking sheet for 2 minutes after removal from oven and then move to complete cooling on wire rack. Serve as is or ice as desired.

22. What is the text structure used in the passage above?

    (A) sequence
    (B) cause–effect
    (C) comparison–contrast
    (D) description

23. What is word is created by following the directions below?

    Begin with N V R S.

    1. Add C to the beginning of the letter sequence.
    2. Add E before R and after S.
    3. Add O after C.

    (A) co-create
    (B) converse
    (C) creatures
    (D) converted

24. Follow the directions to determine your final location. All roads are North-South or East-West. How is the final destination related to the starting point?

    Step 1. Travel west on Americas Drive.
    Step 2. Turn left on Universe Blvd.
    Step 3. Turn right on Ohio St.
    Step 4. Turn left on Ontario Rd.
    Step 5. Travel 10 miles and turn left on Erie Lane.
    Step 6. End at 200 Erie Lane.

    (A) East
    (B) South
    (C) North
    (D) West

```
1 tbsp yeast

1 1/3 cup milk

1 tsp sugar

2 1/3 cup almond flour

2 tsp xanthan gum

1 tsp salt

2 tsp olive oil

2 tsp cider vinegar

1/3 cup corn meal
```

25. The above recipe would provide for which special dietary need?

   (A) gluten intolerance
   (B) glucose intolerance
   (C) lactose intolerance
   (D) corn allergy

26. The consumption of lead (1) can **lead** (2) to blood and brain disorders. What is the meaning of *lead* (2) in this sentence?

   (A) a clue
   (B) to induce
   (C) a forerunner
   (D) to be in charge

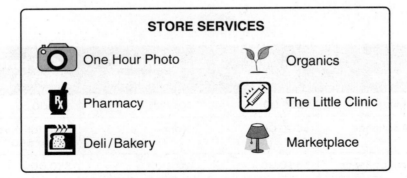

27. A four-year-old child needs age appropriate immunizations. According to the above, which area of the store would be the most likely department to visit?

   (A) deli/bakery
   (B) organics
   (C) The Little Clinic
   (D) pharmacy

28. According to the above table of contents, on which page of this book would you find information on estimating costs based on safety concerns?

    (A) 94

    (B) 74

    (C) 32

    (D) 28

STORE	COST	ONLINE COUPON	SHIPPING AND INSTALLATION
ABC Hardware	$525.00	10% off	$75.00
CostSav Appliance	$600.00	None	Free for purchase above $500.00
YourHome Appliance	$600.00	20% off	$50.00
Home Appliance	$475.00	None	$95.00

29. Which of the above providers offers the most reasonable cost for the appliance?

    (A) YourHome

    (B) Home

    (C) CostSav

    (D) ABC

30. A chef wants to learn more about the nutritional value of polenta. Which online source would be most trustworthy?

(A) Food and Drug Administration
(B) Health and Happiness
(C) Self Nutrition
(D) Your Nutrition Labels

31. You are planning a party and must give specific instructions regarding the seating and table locations. Your party room is 20 feet long and 15 feet wide. Tables are 5 feet in diameter (with comfortable seating extending out to 2 feet from the edge of the table) and comfortably seat as many as 6 per table. How many people can you invite if you maximize the space?

(A) 48
(B) 42
(C) 36
(D) 24

32. The teacher wanted to **record** a high grade in the student record but was held to ethical standards. What is the meaning of the bolded word in the sentence above?

(A) a document
(B) a testimony
(C) to log
(D) to tape

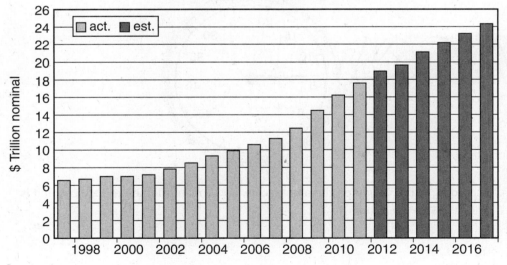

Gross Public Dept
US from FY 1997 to FY 2017

33. According to the graph, actual debt increased the most in which year?

(A) 2000
(B) 2003
(C) 2009
(D) 2013

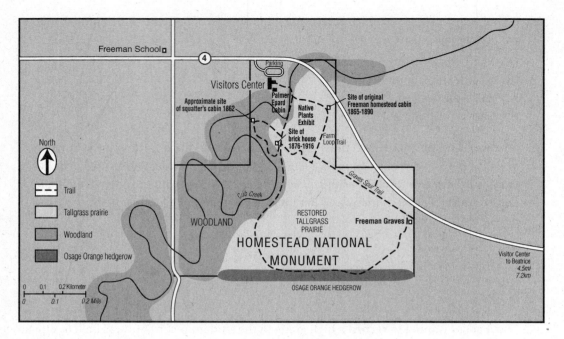

34. According to the map, what would be the shortest route from the parking area to the brick house?

   (A) the walking path that passes the squatter's cabin
   (B) the walking path that passes the original homestead cabin
   (C) the walking path that passes the freeman school
   (D) the walking path that passes the native plants display

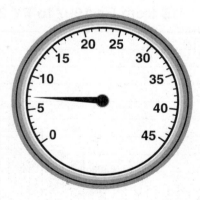

35. According to the weight on the above scale, how much will the produce cost if it is priced at $2.95 per pound?

   (A) $20.65
   (B) $19.20
   (C) $17.70
   (D) $15.25

```
┌─────────────────────────────────┐
│ Scenic Road Trips               │
│                                 │
│ A.  Across bridges              │
│ B.  Along coastlines            │
│ C.  Through valleys             │
│ D.  Within city limits          │
└─────────────────────────────────┘
```

36. For the above table of contents, which topic would best fit as the next logical section of this book?

    (A) Within a garden

    (B) Between borders

    (C) With friends

    (D) On a cruise

Test dates for pre-entrance exams

January 31 in Lakeview

February 24 in Gushton

March 12 and 25 in Ashville

April 2 and 15 in Titan

Enroll online for your preferred test date. You must register one week before the exam. You will not be seated for the exam if you register late.

---

37. According to the above schedule, if you want to take the exam in Ashville and you are working on March 25, when is the last possible date to register?

    (A) March 8

    (B) February 25

    (C) March 5

    (D) February 31

Deductions

Earnings	$1036.00
Federal Income Tax	$102.18
Social Security Tax	$50.20
Medicare Tax	$15.02

38. Based on the table, what percentage is being deducted from this paycheck for Social Security Tax?

    (A) between 0 and 1%

    (B) between 2 and 5%

    (C) between 6 and 7.5%

    (D) between 10 and 15%

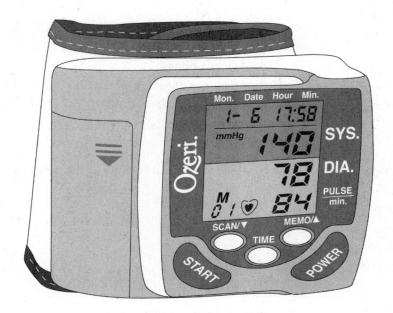

39. Based on the above figure, what is the pulse rate?

(A) 78

(B) 84

(C) 140

(D) 175

40. A student wants to improve an achievement test score on the second attempt. What is the best resource?

(A) study guide/review book

(B) classroom notes

(C) instructor advice

(D) encyclopedia

Textbook Section Listing	
a. Computers and the Professional	1–38
b. Computer Systems	39–45
c. International Perspectives	46–65
d. The Future of Informatics	66–110

41. Based on the above table of contents, where would the chapter on the use of computer hardware be located?

(A) pages 1–38

(B) pages 39–45

(C) pages 46–65

(D) pages 66–110

QUESTIONS 42 AND 43 ARE BASED ON THE FOLLOWING ANNOUNCEMENT.

By clicking the button you agree that we may contact you at the above-listed phone number with a pre-recorded message to verify your interest in receiving quotes. You will have the opportunity to opt out of receiving future pre-recorded messages. You consent to receive autodialed calls, e-mails, and text messages from or on behalf of agents and carriers at the telephone number and e-mail address you provided above. Receiving quotes through our website is always free and you are under no obligation to purchase any goods or services as a result of this request. You understand that consent is not a condition of purchase and you may also receive a quote by contacting us via phone.

42. In the above passage, what is the reason for the hyphen in *pre-recorded*?

   (A) to write a compound word
   (B) to draw attention to the phrase
   (C) to identify modifiers
   (D) to divide

43. What is the purpose of the passage above?

   (A) to be a disclaimer
   (B) to obtain a quote
   (C) to oblige you to purchase
   (D) to obtain consent

We noticed you haven't uploaded anything to your account yet. Once you've uploaded, you can stream music and videos to your mobile device, store and access your files securely, and share files with friends and family easily and privately.

Uploading is easy: just drag and drop. So what are you waiting for? Visit the site today to get started!

Need help uploading? Check out our product page.

Your Online Team.

---

44. What is the purpose of the above e-mail message?

   (A) to persuade
   (B) to inform
   (C) to entertain
   (D) to express feelings

QUESTIONS 45 AND 46 ARE BASED ON THE FOLLOWING PASSAGE.

Mindful Dieting

Magic pills, liquid diets, compulsive exercising... sound familiar? Many people who want to lose weight are often tempted by the latest fad. Problem is, the weight lost with these "quick fixes" can be expensive and often doesn't last. Instead, get results by using something you already have—your mind!

Okay, that may sound a little new-agey. But the truth is mindfulness could be the key to your weight loss success. Being mindful simply means to give your full attention to your environment, thoughts, behaviors, and experiences.

(Retrieved from: http://www.webmd.com/diet/)

45. What is the author's purpose for writing this article about weight loss?

   (A) to entertain the reader
   (B) to express feelings
   (C) to inform the reader
   (D) to persuade the reader

46. What is the purpose of the dash in "have—your mind" in the above passage?

   (A) to replace a colon
   (B) to work like a parenthesis
   (C) to emphasize a series of information
   (D) to add more information at the end of a sentence

QUESTIONS 47 AND 48 ARE BASED ON THE FOLLOWING PASSAGE.

The team then showed forty-eight undergraduate students the first photo for one and a half seconds, followed by a one-second pause, before revealing the other photo. Participants then had to indicate if there were any differences between the photos and, if so, what those differences were. (The students could pick possible changes from a list.)

Participants often accurately detected there were changes in the photos. But the students weren't very good at identifying what had changed, even with big alterations, such as the removal of a large Mexican hat. The same phenomenon is at play when friends miss that new hairstyle or pair of glasses, or sense a change but can't quite put their finger on it.

47. Which type of literature is this passage most likely from?

   (A) textbook
   (B) science fiction novel
   (C) research journal
   (D) mystery novel

48. What is the author most likely addressing in this article?

   (A) déjà vu
   (B) memory
   (C) vision
   (D) sixth sense

Part 2: Mathematics

Time: 51 minutes

34 questions

1. Simplify the expression: $(6 \times 3) \div (8 \times 5)$.

   (A) 0.54
   (B) 3.20
   (C) 0.45
   (D) 1.16

2. Simplify the expression: $-3(5-9+4)$.

   (A) 2
   (B) 24
   (C) -24
   (D) 0

3. Simplify the expression: $1.354 - 0.982$.

   (A) 3.720
   (B) -372
   (C) 1.273
   (D) 0.372

4. Simplify the expression: $0.367 - 4.233$.

   (A) 5.8037
   (B) -3.866
   (C) -4.2687
   (D) 3.866

•A_____•B_____•C

5. In the diagram above, the distance between A and B is 12 feet, and the distance between B and C is the distance between A and B multiplied by 5.

   What is the distance between B and C?

   (A) 15
   (B) 60
   (C) 17
   (D) 56

6. A pharmacist is to reconstitute a powdered drug by adding a specific amount of milliliters (ml) of sterile water per vial; available are two options: 500-milligram (mg) vials and 1-gram (g) vials. The instructions read, "Add 10 ml of sterile water to the 500-mg vial or 20 ml to the 1-g vial of dry, sterile powder." If the pharmacist reconstitutes five 500-mg vials, how many ml of sterile water will be used to reconstitute all five vials?

   (A) 10
   (B) 100
   (C) 50
   (D) 20

7. What is the sum of $6\frac{2}{3}+2\frac{1}{4}$?

   (A) $\frac{100}{12}$
   (B) $8\frac{11}{12}$
   (C) $8\frac{5}{6}$
   (D) $5\frac{6}{7}$

8. What is the quotient of $5\frac{5}{4}\div\frac{2}{5}$?

   (A) $15\frac{3}{7}$
   (B) $15\frac{5}{8}$
   (C) 2
   (D) $10\frac{1}{2}$

9. What is the product of $0.25\times\frac{2}{7}$?

   (A) 1.13
   (B) 0.92
   (C) 0.875
   (D) 0.071

10. Which of the following decimals is an approximate equivalent to $\sqrt{17}$?

   (A) 4.123
   (B) 5.001
   (C) 3.899
   (D) 2.936

11. A market value decreases from 257 to 123. What is the percent decrease?

   (A) 45
   (B) 65
   (C) 209
   (D) 52

12. Convert 0.0725 to a percent.

    (A) 7.25%

    (B) 0.75%

    (C) 72.5%

    (D) 0.07%

13. Which of the following rational numbers is greater?

    (A) 0.559

    (B) 4/7

    (C) 0.563

    (D) 5/9

14. Estimate the solution to $374,325 - 27,625$.

    (A) 401,950

    (B) 238,817

    (C) 346,700

    (D) 399,580

15. Reconcile this savings account for this month. The previous balance was $3,525.55. Deposits were made for $2,125.42 and $150.25, and there is a service charge of $7. Withdrawals were made for $1,500 and $599. What is the balance after reconciling this account?

    (A) $6,907.22

    (B) $3,225.59

    (C) $5,625.50

    (D) $2,732.75

16. An employee earns $25 per hour. Deductions for each weekly pay period include: $161.12 taxes, $55.13 medical insurance, and $30.25 retirement. If the employee works five 8-hour shifts each week, what is the take-home pay each week?

    (A) $753.50

    (B) $998.35

    (C) $659.25

    (D) $840.55

17. A student is buying books and supplies for the semester. A lab coat is $25.25, a textbook is $198.95, a study guide is $52.22, and a computer gadget is $56.29. What is the total cost of these purchases?

    (A) $233.17

    (B) $332.71

    (C) $355.29

    (D) $245.51

18. A catered dining event is planned for 52 people. The catering agency charges the following per person: $2.29 per appetizer, $5.25 for a mixed vegetable entrée, $7.55 for a meat entrée with two vegetables, $3.25 for dessert, and $2.17 for a drink. Twenty-one people select the vegetable entrée, and the rest choose the meat entrée. If everyone is served an appetizer, a dessert, and a drink, what is the total price of this event?

(A) $855.52
(B) $351.01
(C) $745.22
(D) $392.60

19. A graduating chef student is preparing a mixture from an assortment of spices labeled by color; the mixture requires 2/5 tsp of red, 3/4 tsp of yellow, 5/7 tsp of green, and 1/4 tsp brown. How many total teaspoons will be used in the final mixture?

(A) 3.2
(B) 1.7
(C) 2.9
(D) 2.1

20. The 25 students that scored a C in a test make up 70% of the students in the class. What is the total number of students in this class?

(A) 35
(B) 45
(C) 55
(D) 30

21. The number of students to clinical faculty in a nursing school cannot exceed 12 students per 1 instructor. How many instructors will be needed for a group of 60 students?

(A) 7
(B) 4
(C) 6
(D) 5

22. What is 1999 in Roman numerals?

(A) IXXXCIX
(B) IX-XCIX
(C) MCMXCIX
(D) MDCCCCX

23. An antique gold coin was found stamped with the date MCLVI. What is this date in conventional numbers?

(A) 1154
(B) 1156
(C) 1301
(D) 1056

24. How many feet are in 10 meters?

 (A) 25
 (B) 29
 (C) 33
 (D) 35

25. A weight-loss customer was told to reach an ideal weight of 77 kilograms. What is the approximate equivalent in pounds?

 (A) 120
 (B) 140
 (C) 170
 (D) 155

26. A manufacturing inspector needs to verify the dimensions of a 3-inch tool for precision. What measuring tool would be most appropriate?

 (A) caliper
 (B) ruler
 (C) graded cylinder
 (D) fine scales

27. The scale on a blueprint of a house assigns 1 inch to 5 feet. If a room shows a length of $2\frac{1}{4}$ inches and a width of $1\frac{1}{8}$ inches, what are the actual dimensions of the room?

 (A) $12\frac{1}{8}\times7\frac{1}{2}$ feet
 (B) $11\frac{1}{4}\times5\frac{5}{8}$ feet
 (C) $10\frac{1}{4}\times4\frac{1}{8}$ feet
 (D) $14\frac{1}{4}\times12\frac{1}{8}$ feet

28. In the sentence, "Bad company corrupts good manners," which is the dependent variable?

 (A) bad
 (B) company
 (C) corrupts
 (D) manners

**Favorite Lunch Food of
High School Students**

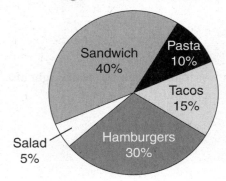

29. According to the above graph, how many students would prefer hamburgers for lunch from a sample of 100 students?

    (A) 10
    (B) 15
    (C) 30
    (D) 40

30. Of the following graph types, which would best represent changes over a period of time?

    (A) bar
    (B) circle
    (C) line
    (D) histogram

31. Simplify the expression: $(7x^2 + 6x - 9) - (x^2 - 8x - 2)$.

    (A) $3x^2 + 2x - 6$
    (B) $6x^2 + 14x - 7$
    (C) $3x(2x - 2)$
    (D) $5x^2 + x - 5$

32. Express the following case in mathematical form: Dan's sister is 3 years less than the sum of their ages and 2; if the sum of their ages is f, how old is she?

    (A) $f - 1 = x$
    (B) $f - 3 = x$
    (C) $f + 2 = x$
    (D) $-f + 5 = x$

33. Solve this equation for k: $k - 4 = 9$.

   (A) 9
   (B) 13
   (C) 11
   (D) 7

34. Solve the inequality: $|2x - 3| > 7$.

   (A) $x < -2$ and $x > 5$
   (B) $x < -4$ and $x > 10$
   (C) $x < -2$ or $x > 5$
   (D) $x < +2$ or $x > -5$

Part 3: Science

Time: 66 minutes
54 questions

QUESTIONS 1 AND 2 ARE BASED ON THE FOLLOWING PERIODIC TABLE.

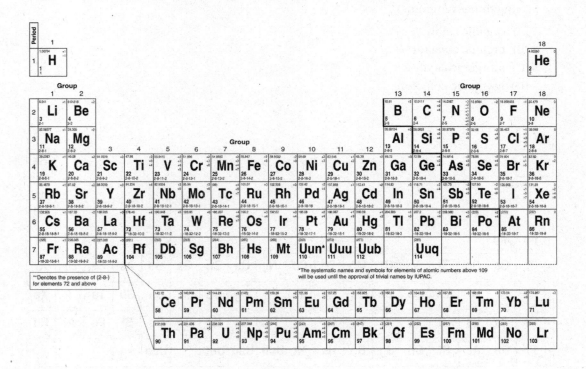

1. How many neutrons and electrons are present in a neutral isotope of copper (Cu)?
   (Atomic weight is 63.55.)

   (A) 8 electrons and 8 neutrons
   (B) 10 electrons and 15 neutrons
   (C) 30 electrons and 30 neutrons
   (D) 29 electrons and 35 neutrons

2. Which elements are most similar in reactivity?

   (A) H and He
   (B) Li and Be
   (C) Mg and Ca
   (D) Zn and Ag

3. Which of the following devices does NOT utilize radio waves?

 (A) television remote control
 (B) cellular telephone
 (C) satellite
 (D) radar

4. When an object is thrown up into the air, its velocity continues to decrease. What happens to the kinetic energy when the velocity becomes zero?

 (A) The law of conservation of energy takes over.
 (B) It becomes potential.
 (C) It remains kinetic.
 (D) The energy decreases to 50%.

5. What is the name of the cofactor that contains carbon and hydrogen and is made from living things (vitamins) ?

 (A) organic catalyst
 (B) organic cofactor
 (C) inorganic catalyst
 (D) inorganic cofactor

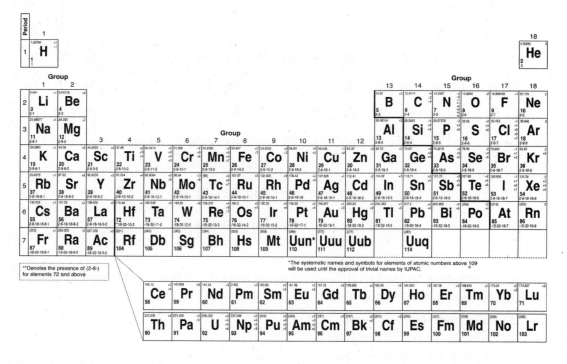

6. According to the above periodic table, what happens as you move from top to bottom?

 (A) electronegativity decreases
 (B) electronegativity increases
 (C) ionization energy decreases
 (D) ionization energy increases

7. The noble gases, in the farthest right column of the periodic chart, have which chemical property as a group?

   (A) They want to gain one electron to develop a full electron outer shell.
   (B) They have a high conductivity.
   (C) They are highly reactive.
   (D) They have a low electron affinity because of the full outer shell.

8. A client has been told to decrease intake of acid drinks. Which beverage would be lowest in pH?

   (A) water
   (B) orange juice
   (C) milk
   (D) green tea

9. Where are hydrocarbons found in nature?

   (A) in inorganic substances
   (B) within living substances
   (C) in oxygen tanks
   (D) dissolved in water only

10. Which column of the periodic table contains the elements most likely to share bonds of electronegativity?

    (A) nonmetal
    (B) noble gases
    (C) metalloids
    (D) alkali metals

11. How many molecules of Na_2S will you have in this equation once it is balanced?
    __ AgI + __ Na_2S → __ Ag_2S + __ NaI

    (A) 1
    (B) 2
    (C) 3
    (D) 5

12. Why is water essential for metabolic processes?

    (A) It is the universal solute.
    (B) It participates in anabolism and catabolism.
    (C) It has high vaporization.
    (D) It forms the standard for the freezing point.

13. What is the difference between a solid and liquid in properties?

    (A) Liquid molecules do not move.
    (B) Solid molecules are easily compressed.
    (C) Liquid molecules assume the shape of their container.
    (D) There is lots of free space between liquid molecules.

14. Which rewording of this hypothesis will make it more directional and better defined? "The community leaders noticed that the citizens of the town are gaining weight and becoming out of physical conditioning."

(A) There is a relationship between availability of healthy food and body weight of the people of this town.
(B) If the people stop eating they will lose weight.
(C) Less public transportation will decrease the weight of people in this town.
(D) Teaching about calories should make a real difference.

15. What is the research focus of this statement? "Pets who receive more attention from humans are of a greater than normal body weight."

(A) directional hypothesis
(B) non-directional hypothesis
(C) a research argument
(D) not a researchable problem as stated

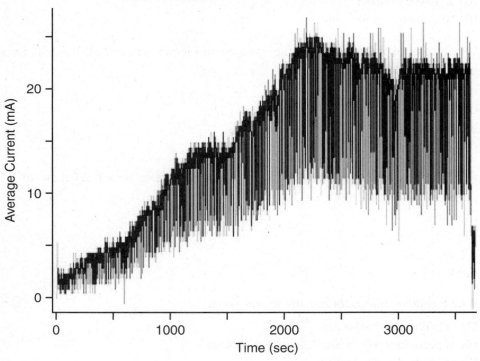

Copper Nanowires Covered with Aluminum

16. The above graph is a data collection done over time to determine the strength of a certain type of wiring to be used for electronic devices. This was presented recently in a team meeting for discussion. What phase of the research process is the team approaching?

(A) question asking
(B) data collection
(C) analysis
(D) conclusion

17. Which research variable(s) is/are involved in a cause-and-effect relationship?

   (A) independent
   (B) dependent
   (C) both independent and dependent
   (D) neither independent nor dependent

18. The study is called: "Is the number of prenatal visits of pregnant women associated with labor and delivery outcomes?" What are the dependent and independent variables?

   (A) visits, women
   (B) pregnancy, delivery
   (C) outcomes, visits
   (D) labor, delivery

19. A researcher goes to a community action group setting to find out about a research topic, and collects data at the site to develop a way to measure the outcomes after the planned intervention. What type of study design is this?

   (A) either qualitative or quantitative
   (B) quantitative
   (C) qualitative
   (D) mixed

20. The researcher discovers a new gadget and wants to get a patent after further trial. What type of reasoning is this?

   (A) quantitative
   (B) deductive
   (C) inductive
   (D) proactive

21. The research team is planning to collect data on a phenomenon from retrospective information. Which of these designs would fit?

   (A) non-experimental design
   (B) qualitative design
   (C) experimental design
   (D) survey

22. The researchers are attempting to formulate scientific model or theory based on mixed data. What would give the highest confidence in a theoretical model?

   (A) There is transferability and reproducibility.
   (B) The model fails the test in one area of the intervention.
   (C) There is a researcher bias.
   (D) The instrument is accurate and reflects the model's assumptions.

23. A researcher is collecting data in a quantitative study on BMI (body mass index) data. Which type of equipment would be needed?

   (A) questionnaire
   (B) audio recorder
   (C) scale with height bar
   (D) telephone

24. In what language is the species biological classification system written?

   (A) English
   (B) Latin
   (C) Greek
   (D) French

25. Why would a group of chickens develop sharper beaks to enable them to eat grains faster?

   (A) competition for food
   (B) competition for shelter
   (C) change in climate
   (D) increase in predators

26. What are the building blocks of proteins called?

   (A) polypeptides
   (B) lipase
   (C) enzymes
   (D) amino acids

27. Which cellular organelle is responsible for the amount of protein in the cell?

   (A) lysosome
   (B) endoplasmic reticulum
   (C) mitochondrion
   (D) Golgi apparatus

28. What happens when a person has an extra chromosome?

   (A) high achievement in school
   (B) Down syndrome
   (C) reddish-brown eyes
   (D) polyracial traits

29. What is the main reason mitosis is important to the organism?

   (A) to replace old cells
   (B) for genetic adaptation
   (C) to allow for replacement of slow growing cells
   (D) to allow for adequate organism reproduction

30. Where are the ribosomes in cells located?

    (A) inside the nucleus
    (B) near the cell membrane
    (C) on the endoplasmic reticulum
    (D) inside a vacuole

31. What principle of Mendelian genetics supports the result of crossing two traits of parents when only one trait appears?

    (A) segregation
    (B) independent assortment
    (C) dominance and recessiveness
    (D) allele frequency

32. What could be considered unique to viruses?

    (A) They contain no DNA or RNA.
    (B) They can reproduce independently.
    (C) They can replicate in a host cell.
    (D) They are easily killed by antibiotics.

33. Which antibody is most abundant in the human body?

    (A) IgG
    (B) IgM
    (C) IgA
    (D) IgE

34. If two parents with red–green color blindness meet, what is the chance their children could be affected with this X-linked recessive trait?

    (A) 25%
    (B) 50%
    (C) 100% all females
    (D) 100% all males

35. Which chamber of the heart receives blood from the systemic circulation?

    (A) right atrium
    (B) right ventricle
    (C) left atrium
    (D) left ventricle

36. What structure transmits electrical stimulus to the atrioventricular septum?

    (A) SA node
    (B) AV node
    (C) bundle of His
    (D) left ventricle

37. What causes the initiation of a cardiac contraction?

    (A) decreased cell permeability to ions
    (B) rapid movement of ions across the cell membrane
    (C) a blockage of calcium ions
    (D) a stimulus initiated during the refractory period

38. What is the slit-shaped space between the true vocal cords called?

    (A) glottis
    (B) epiglottis
    (C) larynx
    (D) carina

39. What type of membranes surround the lungs?

    (A) mucous
    (B) serous
    (C) synovial
    (D) peritoneal

40. What is the primary function of the pulmonary system?

    (A) intake and expelling of air
    (B) exchange of gases between the environment and blood
    (C) movement of blood into and out of the capillaries
    (D) principle mechanism for cooling of the heart

41. Which of the sweat glands are most abundant in the axilla and genital areas?

    (A) eccrine
    (B) apocrine
    (C) sebaceous
    (D) subcutaneous

42. What is the functional unit of the kidney?

    (A) calyx
    (B) nephron
    (C) collecting duct
    (D) pyramid

43. Which nephrons determine the concentration of the urine?

    (A) juxtamedullary
    (B) juxtacortical
    (C) cortical
    (D) medullary

44. Which nephron accounts for 85% of all nephrons?

    (A) juxtamedullary
    (B) juxtacortical
    (C) cortical
    (D) medullary

45. How much cardiac output is supplied to the kidneys on average?

    (A) 10% to 20%
    (B) 15% to 20%
    (C) 20% to 25%
    (D) 30% to 35%

46. Which area of the brain could be treated by a sleeping medication for insomnia?

    (A) corpora quadrigemina
    (B) reticular activating system
    (C) cerebellum
    (D) hypothalamus

47. What are the convolutions on the surface of the cerebrum called?

    (A) sulci
    (B) fissures
    (C) reticular formations
    (D) gyri

48. What is the region responsible for motor aspects of speech termed?

    (A) Wernicke area
    (B) Broca area
    (C) primary speech area
    (D) insula

49. Where is the vermiform appendix attached?

    (A) duodenum
    (B) ileum
    (C) cecum
    (D) sigmoid colon

50. What change in the body can trigger antidiuretic hormone (ADH) release from the posterior pituitary?

    (A) low blood pressure sensed by baroreceptors in the kidneys
    (B) high serum osmolarity sensed by osmoreceptors in the hypothalamus
    (C) low osmolarity sensed by osmoreceptors in the kidneys
    (D) high concentration of potassium sensed by chemoreceptors in the carotid body

51. What mechanism is used by many target cells to adapt to high hormone levels?

    (A) negative feedback
    (B) positive feedback
    (C) down-regulation
    (D) up-regulation

52. What is an essential ingredient for thyroid hormone synthesis?

    (A) zinc
    (B) sodium
    (C) iodine
    (D) calcium

53. What are the most abundant cells in the blood?

    (A) leukocytes
    (B) lymphocytes
    (C) erythrocytes
    (D) thrombocytes

54. Plasma proteins synthesized by lymphocytes in the lymph nodes are:

    (A) globulins
    (B) albumins
    (C) clotting factors
    (D) complement proteins

Part 4: English and Language Usage

Time: 34 minutes

34 questions

1. Bill and Bob, while visiting grandma _____ , stayed in touch with mom.

   Which of the following options correctly completes the sentence above?

   (A) fanciful
   (B) frantic
   (C) faithfully
   (D) frequent

2. <u>The</u> boy <u>who played harder</u> tired first.

   Which of the following correctly identifies the parts of speech in the underlined portions of the sentence above?

   (A) subject; adverb
   (B) pronoun; object
   (C) adjective; clause
   (D) article; clause

3. Which of the following sentences has correct subject–verb agreement?

   (A) When they often visit a new restaurant, he always finds the restroom first.
   (B) The reunion seldom linger, the family then retreats for the day.
   (C) When I yearningly want silence, the neighbor only give me mayhem.
   (D) The club seems impartial until it only admit their own.

4. Which of the following sentences provides an example of correct subject–verb agreement?

   (A) The faculty, upon analyzing applicant records, accepts only the top one hundred.
   (B) The crowd, pleased with the show, cheer until the band comes back.
   (C) The team of participants are performing in orchestrated harmony.
   (D) The group of cyclists, viewing the intricate map, choose the alternate trail.

5. Todd and <u>Muffy</u> chose to return on separate hiking routes. He began to worry when it was taking longer for ___ to come back.

   Which of the following options is the correct pronoun for the sentence above? The antecedent of the pronoun to be added is underlined

   (A) they
   (B) us
   (C) she
   (D) her

6. We took a stroll with newcomers Al and Abby at the nearby park; while enjoying the scenery, people ignored us but befriended ___.

   Which of the following is the correct pronoun to complete the sentence above?

   (A) we
   (B) us
   (C) them
   (D) they

7. Which is an example of a correctly punctuated direct dialogue sentence?

   (A) Loni asked me, How far "do you" want to go?
   (B) "How far do you want to go?" Loni asked me.
   (C) "How far do you want to go"? she asked me.
   (D) How far, she asked me, do you want to go.

8. Which sentences are correctly punctuated for direct dialogue?

   (A) Susan confided, "I'd rather read 'fiction' over any other 'literary' style."
   (B) I'd rather read fiction over any other literary style, confided Susan.
   (C) "Over any other literary style," confided Susan, "I'd rather read fiction."
   (D) Susan confided that "she'd rather read fiction over any other literary style."

9. Which of the following is an example of second-person point of view?

   (A) They suggested me to leave the concert toward the start of the last song to avoid the heavy traffic.
   (B) To avoid the heavy traffic Fay and I wanted to leave the concert when the last song started.
   (C) To avoid the heavy traffic, Gail and Bryan agreed to leave the concert when the last song started.
   (D) Lana and you must decide to leave the concert before the last song to avoid the heavy traffic.

10. Which of the following sentences in the instructions below is an example of second-person voice?

    (A) As soon as you see the curve, make a right and then a quick left turn.
    (B) Once anyone sees the curve, it is easy to make the right and quick left turns.
    (C) As soon as I missed the curve, there was no way to turn right and then left.
    (D) After we saw the curve, we failed to see the way to turn right and then left.

11. Ed and Edna played tennis. The rain started. He wanted to play table tennis. She went shopping.

    Which option best uses grammar for style and clarity to combine the sentences above?

    (A) Ed and Edna played tennis when the rain started; he wanted to play table tennis, and she went shopping.
    (B) While Ed and Edna played tennis, the rain started; he wanted to play table tennis while she went shopping.
    (C) The rain started while Ed and Edna played tennis; he wanted to play table tennis, but she went shopping.
    (D) The rain started while they played tennis; Edna went shopping while Ed wanted to play table tennis.

12. We went to the springs. The waters were deep. The day was dawning. We plunged in.

   Which option best uses grammar for style and clarity to combine the sentences above?

   (A) We went to the springs, the waters were deep and the day was dawning, so we plunged in.
   (B) When we went to the springs, the waters were deep; however, since the day was dawning, we plunged in.
   (C) When we went to the springs, the waters were deep; since the day was dawning, we plunged in.
   (D) The waters were deep when we went to the springs, but we plunged in because the day was dawning.

13. In their raiding path, they left every business place rifled.

   Which of the following is the meaning of the word *rifled* as used in the sentence above?

   (A) plundered
   (B) gun-fired
   (C) demolished
   (D) unscathed

14. His brave actions belied his constant doubts and fears.

   Which of the following is the meaning of the word *belied*?

   (A) endured
   (B) revealed
   (C) discovered
   (D) contradicted

15. No offer followed the interview, and eventually an insider confided that the decision was predetermined.

   In the sentence above, the prefix *pre-* indicates that the situation was related to what type of instance?

   (A) decided instead
   (B) decided before
   (C) decided afterwards
   (D) decided in haste

16. The new teacher tended to speak within the tenets of globalism.

   In the sentence above, the suffix *–ism* in *globalism* can best be defined by which of the following words?

   (A) state or condition
   (B) having to do with
   (C) belief in
   (D) study of

17. Which of the following words is spelled correctly?

   (A) annoyence
   (B) baggage
   (C) consciencious
   (D) divisable

18. Which of the following words is spelled correctly?

    (A) mimicked
    (B) emergencie
    (C) prosetion
    (D) slieght

19. He had chronic _____ so reading the adventure story gave no relief to his wakefulness.

    Which option correctly completes the sentence above?

    (A) somnolence
    (B) depression
    (C) insomnia
    (D) tedium

20. If they'd been _____, we'd be in the next town _____.

    Which option correctly completes the question above?

    (A) all ready; allready
    (B) all ready; already
    (C) already; all-ready
    (D) already; allreddy

21. With them, they had no small <u>dissencion</u> and disputation.

    Which word corrects the spelling of the underlined word to the sentence above?

    (A) discension
    (B) dicenssion
    (C) dicention
    (D) dissention

22. Which of the following underlined words is an example of correct spelling?

    (A) Because her hair took longer in <u>dying</u>, her beautician kept her longer.
    (B) Her unconventional <u>genera</u> of novel writing was puzzling.
    (C) Because of the <u>stationery</u> nature of the road, he arrived late to the meeting.
    (D) Unlike your usual tardiness, <u>you're</u> here early today.

23. Which of the following sentences follows the rules of capitalization?

    (A) I like the month of June.
    (B) I am with uncle Pete.
    (C) I am from the old South.
    (D) I'll be back in Spring.

24. When we visit China, we'd like to contemplate the Great Wall and a grand scale traditional Chinese garden, such as the water wonderland beauty of west Lake in Hangzhou. Which of the following words in the sentence above should be capitalized?

    (A) grand
    (B) scale
    (C) garden
    (D) west

25. Which of the following sentences correctly applies the rules of punctuation?

    (A) Sheila is very bright, without pretension she is beautiful too.
    (B) Sheila is very bright without pretension; she is beautiful, too.
    (C) Sheila is very bright; without pretension, she is beautiful too.
    (D) Sheila is very bright without pretension: she is beautiful too.

26. No matter how much I tried, I could not sleep at all last night __ I was too involved in my writing project, which is due in a week.

    Which of the following punctuation marks correctly completes the sentence above?

    (A) –
    (B) ,
    (C) ;
    (D) :

27. Which of the following is an example of a simple sentence?

    (A) Alice reads all the time, consistently, and studies every day.
    (B) Alice reads all the time, and tries consistently to study every day.
    (C) Alice reads all the time, but tries to study consistently every day.
    (D) Alice reads all the time, and consistently tries to study every day.

28. Which of the following is an example of a simple sentence?

    (A) The dog of the fluffy waggling tail had barked at the passerby joggers for the last half-hour, but he quieted down when I walked him to my mile-away friends.
    (B) The dog of the fluffy waggling tail had barked at the passerby joggers for the last half-hour, though I walked him to my mile-away friends.
    (C) The dog of the fluffy waggling tail had barked at the passerby joggers for the last half-hour but quieted down with a walk to my mile-away friends.
    (D) The dog of the fluffy waggling tail had barked at the passerby joggers for the last half-hour until I walked him to my mile-away friends.

29. The visitors watched the fireworks. They were fascinated by the glittering display.

    Which of the following uses a conjunction to combine the sentences above so that the focus is more on the visitors' watching of the fireworks and less on their fascination?

    (A) The visitors watched the fireworks; they were fascinated by the glittering display.
    (B) The visitors watched the fireworks and were fascinated by the glittering display.
    (C) The visitors watched the fireworks, and they were fascinated by the glittering display.
    (D) The visitors watched the fireworks, since they were fascinated by the glittering display.

30. The successful students in this program _____

    Which of the following allows the above sentence to be completed as a simple sentence?

    (A) do all their course assignments and usually stay on track.
    (B) do all their course assignments, and manage to stay on track.
    (C) require no further advising, though some skip review sessions.
    (D) require no further advising once they attend all review sessions.

31. Which of the following sentences is most clear and correct?

   (A) Whenever circumstances, right again they return.
   (B) They return whenever circumstances are right.
   (C) Whenever they return, circumstances are right.
   (D) They return right, circumstances are whenever.

32. He said to wait. We sat in suspense. We saw him last. He stumbled away.

   To improve sentence fluency, which of the following best states the information above in a single sentence?

   (A) When he said to wait and we saw him last, he stumbled away as we sat in suspense.
   (B) We saw him last as he said to wait and he stumbled away, as we sat in suspense.
   (C) When he said to wait, we sat in suspense and saw him last as he stumbled away.
   (D) As he stumbled away, we saw him last and he said to wait and we sat in suspense.

33. Gail planted a fruit tree. It was in her backyard. Only grass grew there. It was small.

   To improve sentence fluency, which of the following best states the information above in a single sentence?

   (A) Gail planted a fruit tree in her backyard where only grass grew; it was small.
   (B) A fruit tree in Gail's grass-only backyard was planted when it was small.
   (C) Gail planted a small fruit tree in her backyard where only grass grew.
   (D) Having planted a small fruit tree, only grass grew in Gail's backyard.

34. She wanted to be followed. She drove fast. I lingered behind. I lost sight of her.

   To improve sentence fluency, which of the following best states the information above in a single sentence?

   (A) I lingered behind because she wanted to be followed, she drove fast, and I lost sight of her.
   (B) Because she wanted to be followed and drove fast, I lingered behind and lost sight of her.
   (C) I lost sight of her because she wanted to be followed: she drove fast, and I lingered behind.
   (D) She drove fast, and wanted to be followed; I lingered behind and lost sight of her.

ANSWER KEY
Practice Test 4

READING

1.	A	13.	A	25.	A	37.	C
2.	A	14.	B	26.	B	38.	B
3.	D	15.	B	27.	C	39.	B
4.	C	16.	A	28.	C	40.	A
5.	D	17.	D	29.	A	41.	B
6.	D	18.	D	30.	A	42.	A
7.	A	19.	A	31.	D	43.	D
8.	B	20.	D	32.	C	44.	A
9.	B	21.	A	33.	C	45.	C
10.	B	22.	A	34.	D	46.	D
11.	B	23.	B	35.	A	47.	C
12.	D	24.	B	36.	B	48.	D

MATHEMATICS

1.	C	10.	A	19.	D	28.	D
2.	B	11.	D	20.	A	29.	C
3.	D	12.	A	21.	D	30.	C
4.	B	13.	B	22.	C	31.	B
5.	B	14.	C	23.	B	32.	A
6.	C	15.	D	24.	C	33.	B
7.	B	16.	A	25.	C	34.	C
8.	B	17.	B	26.	A		
9.	D	18.	C	27.	B		

SCIENCE

1.	D	15.	B	29.	A	43.	A
2.	C	16.	C	30.	C	44.	C
3.	A	17.	C	31.	C	45.	C
4.	B	18.	C	32.	C	46.	B
5.	B	19.	D	33.	A	47.	D
6.	A	20.	C	34.	D	48.	B
7.	D	21.	A	35.	A	49.	C
8.	B	22.	A	36.	B	50.	B
9.	B	23.	C	37.	B	51.	C
10.	A	24.	B	38.	A	52.	C
11.	A	25.	D	39.	B	53.	C
12.	B	26.	D	40.	B	54.	A
13.	C	27.	B	41.	B		
14.	A	28.	B	42.	B		

ENGLISH AND LANGUAGE USAGE

1.	C	10.	A	19.	C	28.	C
2.	D	11.	C	20.	B	29.	D
3.	A	12.	C	21.	D	30.	A
4.	A	13.	A	22.	D	31.	B
5.	D	14.	D	23.	A	32.	C
6.	C	15.	B	24.	D	33.	C
7.	B	16.	C	25.	B	34.	B
8.	C	17.	B	26.	D		
9.	D	18.	A	27.	A		

ANSWER EXPLANATIONS

Reading

1. **(A)** The title best represents the theme of the passage. The actual content of the passage is primarily about lucid dreams (topic). The main idea is the increased interest in the ability of the person to use the technique.

2. **(A)** This is an expository passage; it explains a subject to enhance the understanding of a particular idea. Narrative writing tells a story. Technical writing usually addresses precise information. Persuasive writing tries to convince the reader to agree with the author.

3. **(D)** This is the general idea expressed by the author. The other choices reflect more incorrect assumptions not expressed in the passage.

4. **(C)** The bias is a negative one about disbelief regarding lucid dreams. The other responses are supporting details of the passage.

5. **(D)** The sentence that most describes the phenomenon of interest is the definition sentence. The other sentences are supporting details or arguments supporting the individual viewpoints rather than describing the phenomenon itself.

6. **(D)** This response best describes the writer's message. The other responses reflect non-specifics and incorrect information not present in the passage. The author limits the effectiveness to only some individuals. Some of the answers imply universal benefits.

7. **(A)** This passage was intended to entertain the reader and to report on a unique event for one person. It would not be included in World News since it is not written as a news article. It includes a human factor. It is not an editorial since it is not expressing an opinion. It is not specific to football.

8. **(B)** This narrative style was intended to tell a story. It did not explain something as an exposition would. Persuasive writing tries to convince the reader to agree with the author. Technical writing usually addresses precise information.

9. **(B)** This is an historical passage and was written at the time of the event. It is not based on any theory or exposition.

10. **(B)** It is the writer's bias or opinion regarding the real winner of the race. Answer A is a stereotype, C is an aspiration of Jack's, and D is a supporting detail.

11. **(B)** This would be a supporting detail for this story. The topic of the story was about a jockey who won a race while unconscious. The theme built up the event so that the reader could enjoy the story but understand that racing is a sport and requires preparation.

12. **(D)** The overall intent of the passage is to express the author's opinion on using organics for makeup. The other answers express emotions and feelings opposite to the statements in the passage.

13. **(A)** The passage seems to be from the new products section of a journal or magazine. The author was not trying to persuade you to purchase something or trying to get you to laugh. Most business articles provide straightforward information.

14. **(B)** It is implied that the reader wants to track progress. The other answers denote a negative impact from the device.

15. **(B)** This article is giving advice to future college students. The message is to not over-shoot the goal, but rather meet expectations for the chosen degree or career. The other statements are incorrect and in opposition to the overall message.

16. **(A)** The overall purpose is to encourage the reader to slow down and enjoy the environment. The other answers are incorrect and reflect the opposite idea than intended by the writer.

17. **(D)** This was written to elicit an emotional response to a famous quote.

18. **(D)** This passage presents a story of suspense and unknown events common in mystery novels. A textbook would have presented only factual information. A science fiction novel would be written about the unknown. A research journal would present facts from an evidence-based project.

19. **(A)** This is most likely taken from a textbook since it is informative in nature. It is probably not from a research journal since there are no reported results of a study.

20. **(D)** The e-mail is definitely written to ask the customer to sign up on a separate site to receive a bonus.

21. **(A)** The author is encouraging the customer to purchase bonus miles and to accumulate them for the next planned trip.

22. **(A)** This is a sequence. The steps are to be completed as listed. A cause–effect would be if the author had described an action and then a result. A description would describe an object or event. In comparison–contrast the author would list different aspects and then describe the aspects of something else.

23. **(B)** Begin with N V R S; Add C to the beginning of the word, C N V S; add E before R and after S to get C N V E R S E; add O after C to spell CONVERSE.

24. **(B)** The directions follow the schematic

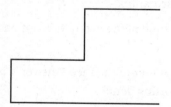

25. **(A)** This recipe has removed all wheat making it ideal for a gluten-free diet. Sugar, milk, and corn meal could be detrimental for others.

26. **(B)** The consumption of *lead* (a metal) *leads* ("induces" or "influences") progression to blood and brain disorders.

27. **(C)** The mother of this child would need to go to The Little Clinic. A health care provider would need to ensure that the immunizations are appropriate before they can be administered.

28. **(C)** The key words "safety" and "estimating costs" point to page 32. Page 94 is the part of the book reviewing safety on the site. Page 74 might mention safety but will not include the key search item. Page 28 is concerned with delivery and estimates and may indirectly mention safety but is not directly addressing the topic.

29. **(A)** 600 – 120 + 50 = 530. All other prices are higher than YourHom when computed from the table: ABC is $547.50; CostSav is $600; and Home is $570.

30. **(A)** The Food and Drug Administration is responsible for protecting our nation's food supply and ensuring honest labeling of foods.

31. **(D)** The room can only accommodate 4 tables with 6 chairs per table, which can accommodate 24 guests overall.

32. **(C)** *Record* is being used as a verb in this sentence; it means "to write down" or "log on a flow sheet."

33. **(C)** 2009 shows an increase of about 2 trillion. The other years demonstrated less than 0.5 trillion, and 2013 is a projected rather than actual increase according to this chart.

34. **(D)** The native plants exhibit is a direct walk from parking to the brick house. The squatter's cabin is a circular drive off to one side of the park. The homestead cabin is far away in another direction from the direct path. The freeman school is outside the park.

35. **(A)** Multiply the scale weight (7 pounds) by 2.95 to get 20.65.

36. **(B)** The outline suggests a distance perspective. "On a cruise" would not be a road trip. "With friends" is another topic not suggested by the title. "A garden" would probably be a walking tour.

37. **(C)** The only date available is March 12 and registration must happen 7 days before the event, so you must register before March 5.

38. **(B)** The deduction is almost 5% since 10% would be 103.6, computed by counting one decimal to the left.

39. **(B)** The pulse is marked as the bottom number on the manometer.

40. **(A)** A study guide is made specifically for the exam and would give more information over a short period of time as compared to the other resources.

41. **(B)** The word *systems* implies equipment and hardware.

42. **(A)** The hyphen enables the author to compound these words.

43. **(D)** The purpose is to obtain the reader's consent for future contacts by the company.

44. **(A)** This e-mail's purpose is to persuade you to upload a program.

45. **(C)** This is written to inform the reader.

46. **(D)** It was used at the end of a sentence to add more information.

47. **(C)** This is a research report. The use of the word *participants* is common in research articles.

48. **(D)** This article is about the possibility of a sixth sense.

Mathematics

1. **(C)** Simplify the expression with the innermost parentheses first. Then work out the rest.

$$\frac{(6\times3)}{(8\times5)}=\frac{18}{40}=0.45$$

2. **(B)** $-3(5-9+4)=-3(5-13)$

$$=-3(-8)$$

$$=24$$

3. **(D)**
$$\begin{array}{r} 1.354 \\ -0.982 \\ \hline 0.372 \end{array}$$

When subtracting whole numbers, numbers are arranged in columns with like place values in each column.

4. **(B)** This option is correct. Thus,

$$\begin{array}{r} 0.367 \\ -4.233 \\ \hline -3.866 \end{array}$$

5. **(B)** This is the only option; thus,

A to B $= 12$

B to C $= 12 \times 5 = 60$.

6. **(C)** Since each 500 mg vial requires 10 ml to be reconstituted, and 5 vials will be used, the total amount of sterile water to be used will be 10 ml × 5 vials = 50 ml.

7. **(B)** First work out the lowest common denominator. Then solve.
$$6\frac{2}{3}+2\frac{1}{4}=\frac{20}{3}+\frac{9}{4}=\frac{80+27}{12}=\frac{107}{12}=8\frac{11}{12}$$

8. **(B)** $\dfrac{\left(5\frac{5}{4}\right)}{\left(\frac{2}{5}\right)}=\dfrac{25}{4}\times\dfrac{5}{2}=\dfrac{125}{8}=15\frac{5}{8}$

Convert the mixed number to an improper fraction. Change the division sign to a multiplication sign and flip the second fraction. Reduce factors in the numerator with factors in the denominator. Then, multiply numerators together and denominators together.

9. **(D)** Convert the fraction to a decimal, and rewrite the given expression accordingly. So,
$.025\times\dfrac{2}{7}= 0.25\times0.285714286 = 0.0714285714$ or 0.071.

10. **(A)** The decimal form 4.123 is greater than the square root of 16 and less than the square root of 25. Since option D is too small, the only option left is A.

11. **(D)** $\dfrac{(257-123)}{257}=52\%$ decrease.

12. **(A)** $0.0725 \times 100 = 7.25\%$

13. **(B)** Convert all numbers to decimals and compare. Since the largest number in the hundredths position is 7, the number 0.571 (converted from $\frac{4}{7}$) is greater than the other numbers.

14. **(C)** Since this is an estimate, start by rounding all integers to easier numbers and compare. So, $400,000 - 30,000 = 370,000$. Because options A and D are too high and option D is too low, the only possible option is C.

15. **(D)** $(3,525.55 + 2,125.42 + 150.25) - (1,500 + 599 + 7) = 5,801.22 - 2106 = \$3,695.22$

16. **(A)** ($1,000 beginning salary) – ($161.12 + 55.13 + 30.25 = \$246.50$ expenses) = \$753.50 left for take-home salary.

17. **(B)** Add all purchased items, thus $25.25 + 198.95 + 52.22 + 56.29 = \$332.71$.

18. **(C)** $(52 \times \$7.71 = \$400.92) + (21 \times \$5.25 = \$110.25) + (31 \times \$7.55 = \$234.05) = \$745.22$

19. **(D)** First find the lowest common denominator. Then solve.

$$\frac{2}{5} + \frac{3}{4} + \frac{5}{7} + \frac{1}{4} = \frac{(56 + 105 + 100 + 35)}{140}$$
$$= \frac{296}{140}$$
$$= 2.114285714 \text{ or } 2.1 \text{ tsp}$$

20. **(A)** If 25 students make up 70% of the class, then 35 students would make up 100% of the class.

21. **(D)** $12x = 60$. Solving by cross-multiplying:

$$x = \frac{60}{12}$$
$$x = 5.$$

22. **(C)** M = 1000, C = 100, X = 10, I = 1. Traditionally, the numbers that follow in decreasing number add to the total number. Thus, M = 1000, CM = 900, XC = 90, IX = 9.

23. **(B)** M = 1000, C = 100, X = 10, V = 5, I = 1. If a smaller number is listed before M, L, X, or V, it will be subtracted from the main number. Traditionally, the numbers that follow in decreasing number add to the total number. Thus, M = 1000, C = 100, L = 50, VI = 6.

24. **(C)** 1 meter = 3.3 feet. Thus, $10 \times 3.3 = 33$ feet.

25. **(C)** 1 kg = 2.2 pounds. Thus, $11 \times 2.2 = 169.4$ or 170.

26. **(A)** Since a length unit is needed to measure a small item, a caliper would be appropriate in this case as these are used to measure lengths smaller than 6 inches with greater precision than a ruler.

27. **(B)** Length is $5 \text{ feet} \times 2\frac{1}{4} \text{ inches} = 11\frac{1}{4}$. Width is $5 \text{ feet} \times 1\frac{1}{8} \text{ inches}$. Thus the room is $11\frac{1}{4}$ feet by $5\frac{5}{8}$ feet.

28. **(D)** The dependent variable is the output based on the input.

29. **(C)** Based on the circle graph data, out of 100 students 30 would prefer to eat hamburgers for lunch.

30. **(C)** A line graph provides a way to show changes over a period of time or compares the relationship between two quantities.

31. **(B)** $(7x^2 + 6x - 9) - (x^2 - 8x - 2) = 6x^2 + 14x - 9 + 2 = 6x^2 + 14x - 7$

32. **(A)** If the sum of their ages is f, and she is $f - 3 + 2$, Dan's sister's age is $x = f - 1$.

33. **(B)** $k - 4 = 9$
$k - 4 + 4 = 9 + 4$
$k = 13$

34. **(C)** $|2x - 3| > 7$

$2x - 3 < -7$ or $2x - 3 > 7$
$2x < -4$ or $2x > 10$
$x < -2$ or $x > 5$

Since there is a lesser than connector, the connecting word is *or*, not *and*.

Science

1. **(D)** The number of electrons is equal to the atomic number; neutrons equal the atomic weight minus the atomic number or number of protons.

2. **(C)** Since they have the same number of electrons available in the outer orbit they are closest in reactivity.

3. **(A)** The television remote control does not use a low-frequency EM wave. It uses infrared waves.

4. **(B)** It becomes potential. Potential energy is stored energy. Kinetic energy is the energy of motion.

5. **(B)** Vitamins are organic cofactors.

6. **(A)** As you move from top to bottom down the periodic table, electronegativity decreases.

7. **(D)** The noble gases, in the farthest right column of the periodic chart, have a full outer electron shell, don't react, and will remain in an oxidative state of 0.

8. **(B)** A client has been told to decrease intake of acid drinks. Orange juice has a pH of 3 to 4; water's pH is 7; milk's is 6.5; and green tea has a pH of 6.5.

9. **(B)** Hydrocarbons are found in living things, foods, fuels, and plastics.

10. **(A)** The nonmetals have the highest propensity to share bonds.

11. **(A)** Balance Ag with 2 for each side. Now you have 2 I so NaI will balance and the others will remain at 1: __ AgI + __ Na_2S → __ Ag_2S + __ NaI.

12. **(B)** Water is involved in catabolism (breaking down of larger molecules and building up) and anabolism.

13. **(C)** Liquids are limited in flow only in volume or containment. They are not easily compressed and the particles can easily slide past one another.

14. **(A)** The statement identifies the problem, suggests a solution, and makes a prediction.

15. **(B)** This is a non-directional hypothesis without a suggested intervention.

16. **(C)** The team is ready to begin the analysis phase of the study.

17. **(C)** Both independent and dependent variables would be included in a cause-and-effect relationship.

18. **(C)** The dependent variable is outcomes, and the independent variable is visits.

19. **(D)** The researcher is mixing methods to get the greatest effect over time.

20. **(C)** Inductive reasoning is taking the idea global.

21. **(A)** Non-experimental designs frequently seek information not to plan to attempt an intervention but just to report on the phenomenon.

22. **(A)** If it were a mixed design, then it would need to meet both tests of validity and reliability for both research methods.

23. **(C)** The data from this study is empirically based and will need a highly reliable instrument for exact measurement.

24. **(B)** This is always written in Latin.

25. **(D)** Increase in predators would create a need for the chickens to be able to eat grains in a sheltered area of the field with harder seeds.

26. **(D)** The building blocks of proteins are amino acids.

27. **(B)** The endoplasmic reticulum moves protein from one part of the cell to another or releases it to the outside of the cell.

28. **(B)** Down syndrome occurs in people with an extra chromosome.

29. **(A)** Mitosis replaces old and dying cells rapidly.

30. **(C)** Ribosomes are located on the endoplasmic reticulum.

31. **(C)** The rule of dominance and recessiveness supports the result of crossing two traits of parents when only one trait appears.

32. **(C)** Viruses can only replicate in their host cells. They either have DNA or RNA. They are not easily killed by antibiotics and are not able to reproduce outside of the host's body.

33. **(A)** IgG is the most common antibody in the human body (70–80%).

34. **(D)** X-linked recessive traits will be carried from mother to son.

35. **(A)** The right atrium receives all venous blood returning from the entire body.

36. **(B)** The AV node continues the electrical conduction originated by the SA node.

37. **(B)** The SA node initiates a rapid movement of ions across the cell membrane.

38. **(A)** The glottis is the slit-shaped space between the true vocal cords. The epiglottis is the small piece of tissue that closes when we swallow.

39. **(B)** A serous membrane surrounds the lungs.

40. **(B)** The lung's primary function is exchange of gases between the environment and blood.

41. **(B)** The apocrine sweat glands are most abundant in the axilla and genitals.

42. **(B)** The nephron is the functional unit of the kidney. The other responses are anatomical structures.

43. **(A)** Juxtamedullary nephrons determine the concentration of the urine.

44. **(C)** Cortical nephrons account for 85% of all nephrons. Juxtamedullary account for about 15%. Cortical nephrons mainly perform excretory and regulatory functions.

45. **(C)** On average, 20 to 25% of cardiac output is supplied to the kidneys.

46. **(B)** The reticular activating system controls sleep.

47. **(D)** The gyri are convolutions on the surface of the cerebrum.

48. **(B)** The Broca area is the region responsible for motor aspects of speech.

49. **(C)** The vermiform appendix is attached to the cecum.

50. **(B)** High serum osmolarity sensed by osmoreceptors in the hypothalamus can trigger antidiuretic hormone (ADH) release from the posterior pituitary.

51. **(C)** Many target cells use down-regulation to adapt to high hormone levels.

52. **(C)** Iodine is an essential ingredient for thyroid hormone synthesis.

53. **(C)** Erythrocytes are the most abundant cells in the blood.

54. **(A)** Globulins are plasma proteins synthesized by lymphocytes in the lymph nodes.

English and Language Usage

1. **(C)** This option contains the proper adjective *faithfully* to complete the sentence. The other options are incorrect in either grammar or case.

2. **(D)** This option correctly identifies *the* as an article and *who played harder* as a clause.

3. **(A)** This option contains correct subject–verb agreement: "they… visit" and "he… finds." All other options contain incorrect subject–verb agreement with regard to number or case.

4. **(A)** This option contains correct subject–verb agreement: "The faculty… accepts." All other options contain incorrect subject–verb agreement with regard to number.

5. **(D)** The antecedent, *Muffy*, is singular and female, which means that *her* is the only correct answer. All other options are incorrect in either number, gender, or case.

6. **(C)** This option completes the sentence as it contains the correct pronoun. All other options are incorrect.

7. **(B)** This option correctly contains double quotation marks around the whole quote. Options A and C contain quotations in the wrong places. Option D has no quotation marks to properly indicate direct dialogue.

8. **(C)** This option correctly contains double quotation marks around the direct quote. Option A unnecessarily adds single quotes, option B has no quotation marks to properly indicate direct dialogue, and option D contains quotations in the wrong places.

9. **(D)** This option is an example of second-person point of view. Options A and C are examples of third-person point of view, and option B is an example of first-person point of view.

10. **(A)** This option is an example of second-person point of view. Option B is an example of third-person point of view. Options C and D are examples of first-person point of view.

11. **(C)** This option effectively uses transitional words to combine the sentences into a single sentence to reflect the original meaning of the group of sentences. All other options may lead to confusion of the writer's original intent.

12. **(C)** This option effectively uses transitional words to combine the sentences into a single sentence that still reflects the original meaning of the group of sentences.

13. **(A)** This option rightly and properly defines the word *rifled* (which has nothing to do with rifles or gunshots). All other options are incorrect.

14. **(D)** This option correctly defines the word *belied*. All other options are incorrect.

15. **(B)** The prefix *pre-* originates from the Latin language. The word *predetermined* means "to settle or decide in advance." Therefore, it can be concluded that this person had no chance of being hired.

16. **(C)** The suffix *-ism* originates from the Latin language. The word *globalism* means "belief in worldwide political impact." Therefore, it can be concluded that this teacher was not enthusiastic about local issues.

17. **(B)** *Baggage* is a commonly misspelled word, its root word (*bag*) ends in *g* which must be doubled (to *bagg*) before adding a suffix that begins with a vowel as in *–age*.

18. **(A)** This option alone is spelled correctly. All other options are spelled incorrectly.

19. **(C)** This option contains the correct word that completes the given sentence. The words "no relief to his wakefulness" point to the meaning of *insomnia*.

20. **(B)** This option contains the only word set that completes the given sentence. *All ready* and *already* are commonly misspelled and misused homophone (sound alike) words.

21. **(D)** This option is spelled correctly; *dissension* is a commonly misspelled word. The noun *disputation* ("argument, debate, discussion") offers a cue to identify *dissension* as the correctly spelled word.

22. **(D)** This option is spelled correctly. All other options are commonly misspelled words: *dying* ("about to die") is not *dyeing* ("coloring"), *genera* ("plural of *genus*") is not *genre* ("literary category"), and *stationery* ("desk items") is not *stationary* ("unmoving," as in bad traffic).

Practice
TESTS

ANSWER SHEET
Practice Test 5

PRACTICE TEST 5

READING

1. Ⓐ Ⓑ Ⓒ Ⓓ	13. Ⓐ Ⓑ Ⓒ Ⓓ	25. Ⓐ Ⓑ Ⓒ Ⓓ	37. Ⓐ Ⓑ Ⓒ Ⓓ
2. Ⓐ Ⓑ Ⓒ Ⓓ	14. Ⓐ Ⓑ Ⓒ Ⓓ	26. Ⓐ Ⓑ Ⓒ Ⓓ	38. Ⓐ Ⓑ Ⓒ Ⓓ
3. Ⓐ Ⓑ Ⓒ Ⓓ	15. Ⓐ Ⓑ Ⓒ Ⓓ	27. Ⓐ Ⓑ Ⓒ Ⓓ	39. Ⓐ Ⓑ Ⓒ Ⓓ
4. Ⓐ Ⓑ Ⓒ Ⓓ	16. Ⓐ Ⓑ Ⓒ Ⓓ	28. Ⓐ Ⓑ Ⓒ Ⓓ	40. Ⓐ Ⓑ Ⓒ Ⓓ
5. Ⓐ Ⓑ Ⓒ Ⓓ	17. Ⓐ Ⓑ Ⓒ Ⓓ	29. Ⓐ Ⓑ Ⓒ Ⓓ	41. Ⓐ Ⓑ Ⓒ Ⓓ
6. Ⓐ Ⓑ Ⓒ Ⓓ	18. Ⓐ Ⓑ Ⓒ Ⓓ	30. Ⓐ Ⓑ Ⓒ Ⓓ	42. Ⓐ Ⓑ Ⓒ Ⓓ
7. Ⓐ Ⓑ Ⓒ Ⓓ	19. Ⓐ Ⓑ Ⓒ Ⓓ	31. Ⓐ Ⓑ Ⓒ Ⓓ	43. Ⓐ Ⓑ Ⓒ Ⓓ
8. Ⓐ Ⓑ Ⓒ Ⓓ	20. Ⓐ Ⓑ Ⓒ Ⓓ	32. Ⓐ Ⓑ Ⓒ Ⓓ	44. Ⓐ Ⓑ Ⓒ Ⓓ
9. Ⓐ Ⓑ Ⓒ Ⓓ	21. Ⓐ Ⓑ Ⓒ Ⓓ	33. Ⓐ Ⓑ Ⓒ Ⓓ	45. Ⓐ Ⓑ Ⓒ Ⓓ
10. Ⓐ Ⓑ Ⓒ Ⓓ	22. Ⓐ Ⓑ Ⓒ Ⓓ	34. Ⓐ Ⓑ Ⓒ Ⓓ	46. Ⓐ Ⓑ Ⓒ Ⓓ
11. Ⓐ Ⓑ Ⓒ Ⓓ	23. Ⓐ Ⓑ Ⓒ Ⓓ	35. Ⓐ Ⓑ Ⓒ Ⓓ	47. Ⓐ Ⓑ Ⓒ Ⓓ
12. Ⓐ Ⓑ Ⓒ Ⓓ	24. Ⓐ Ⓑ Ⓒ Ⓓ	36. Ⓐ Ⓑ Ⓒ Ⓓ	48. Ⓐ Ⓑ Ⓒ Ⓓ

MATHEMATICS

1. Ⓐ Ⓑ Ⓒ Ⓓ	10. Ⓐ Ⓑ Ⓒ Ⓓ	19. Ⓐ Ⓑ Ⓒ Ⓓ	28. Ⓐ Ⓑ Ⓒ Ⓓ
2. Ⓐ Ⓑ Ⓒ Ⓓ	11. Ⓐ Ⓑ Ⓒ Ⓓ	20. Ⓐ Ⓑ Ⓒ Ⓓ	29. Ⓐ Ⓑ Ⓒ Ⓓ
3. Ⓐ Ⓑ Ⓒ Ⓓ	12. Ⓐ Ⓑ Ⓒ Ⓓ	21. Ⓐ Ⓑ Ⓒ Ⓓ	30. Ⓐ Ⓑ Ⓒ Ⓓ
4. Ⓐ Ⓑ Ⓒ Ⓓ	13. Ⓐ Ⓑ Ⓒ Ⓓ	22. Ⓐ Ⓑ Ⓒ Ⓓ	31. Ⓐ Ⓑ Ⓒ Ⓓ
5. Ⓐ Ⓑ Ⓒ Ⓓ	14. Ⓐ Ⓑ Ⓒ Ⓓ	23. Ⓐ Ⓑ Ⓒ Ⓓ	32. Ⓐ Ⓑ Ⓒ Ⓓ
6. Ⓐ Ⓑ Ⓒ Ⓓ	15. Ⓐ Ⓑ Ⓒ Ⓓ	24. Ⓐ Ⓑ Ⓒ Ⓓ	33. Ⓐ Ⓑ Ⓒ Ⓓ
7. Ⓐ Ⓑ Ⓒ Ⓓ	16. Ⓐ Ⓑ Ⓒ Ⓓ	25. Ⓐ Ⓑ Ⓒ Ⓓ	34. Ⓐ Ⓑ Ⓒ Ⓓ
8. Ⓐ Ⓑ Ⓒ Ⓓ	17. Ⓐ Ⓑ Ⓒ Ⓓ	26. Ⓐ Ⓑ Ⓒ Ⓓ	
9. Ⓐ Ⓑ Ⓒ Ⓓ	18. Ⓐ Ⓑ Ⓒ Ⓓ	27. Ⓐ Ⓑ Ⓒ Ⓓ	

SCIENCE

1. Ⓐ Ⓑ Ⓒ Ⓓ
2. Ⓐ Ⓑ Ⓒ Ⓓ
3. Ⓐ Ⓑ Ⓒ Ⓓ
4. Ⓐ Ⓑ Ⓒ Ⓓ
5. Ⓐ Ⓑ Ⓒ Ⓓ
6. Ⓐ Ⓑ Ⓒ Ⓓ
7. Ⓐ Ⓑ Ⓒ Ⓓ
8. Ⓐ Ⓑ Ⓒ Ⓓ
9. Ⓐ Ⓑ Ⓒ Ⓓ
10. Ⓐ Ⓑ Ⓒ Ⓓ
11. Ⓐ Ⓑ Ⓒ Ⓓ
12. Ⓐ Ⓑ Ⓒ Ⓓ
13. Ⓐ Ⓑ Ⓒ Ⓓ
14. Ⓐ Ⓑ Ⓒ Ⓓ

15. Ⓐ Ⓑ Ⓒ Ⓓ
16. Ⓐ Ⓑ Ⓒ Ⓓ
17. Ⓐ Ⓑ Ⓒ Ⓓ
18. Ⓐ Ⓑ Ⓒ Ⓓ
19. Ⓐ Ⓑ Ⓒ Ⓓ
20. Ⓐ Ⓑ Ⓒ Ⓓ
21. Ⓐ Ⓑ Ⓒ Ⓓ
22. Ⓐ Ⓑ Ⓒ Ⓓ
23. Ⓐ Ⓑ Ⓒ Ⓓ
24. Ⓐ Ⓑ Ⓒ Ⓓ
25. Ⓐ Ⓑ Ⓒ Ⓓ
26. Ⓐ Ⓑ Ⓒ Ⓓ
27. Ⓐ Ⓑ Ⓒ Ⓓ
28. Ⓐ Ⓑ Ⓒ Ⓓ

29. Ⓐ Ⓑ Ⓒ Ⓓ
30. Ⓐ Ⓑ Ⓒ Ⓓ
31. Ⓐ Ⓑ Ⓒ Ⓓ
32. Ⓐ Ⓑ Ⓒ Ⓓ
33. Ⓐ Ⓑ Ⓒ Ⓓ
34. Ⓐ Ⓑ Ⓒ Ⓓ
35. Ⓐ Ⓑ Ⓒ Ⓓ
36. Ⓐ Ⓑ Ⓒ Ⓓ
37. Ⓐ Ⓑ Ⓒ Ⓓ
38. Ⓐ Ⓑ Ⓒ Ⓓ
39. Ⓐ Ⓑ Ⓒ Ⓓ
40. Ⓐ Ⓑ Ⓒ Ⓓ
41. Ⓐ Ⓑ Ⓒ Ⓓ
42. Ⓐ Ⓑ Ⓒ Ⓓ

43. Ⓐ Ⓑ Ⓒ Ⓓ
44. Ⓐ Ⓑ Ⓒ Ⓓ
45. Ⓐ Ⓑ Ⓒ Ⓓ
46. Ⓐ Ⓑ Ⓒ Ⓓ
47. Ⓐ Ⓑ Ⓒ Ⓓ
48. Ⓐ Ⓑ Ⓒ Ⓓ
49. Ⓐ Ⓑ Ⓒ Ⓓ
50. Ⓐ Ⓑ Ⓒ Ⓓ
51. Ⓐ Ⓑ Ⓒ Ⓓ
52. Ⓐ Ⓑ Ⓒ Ⓓ
53. Ⓐ Ⓑ Ⓒ Ⓓ
54. Ⓐ Ⓑ Ⓒ Ⓓ

ENGLISH AND LANGUAGE USAGE

1. Ⓐ Ⓑ Ⓒ Ⓓ
2. Ⓐ Ⓑ Ⓒ Ⓓ
3. Ⓐ Ⓑ Ⓒ Ⓓ
4. Ⓐ Ⓑ Ⓒ Ⓓ
5. Ⓐ Ⓑ Ⓒ Ⓓ
6. Ⓐ Ⓑ Ⓒ Ⓓ
7. Ⓐ Ⓑ Ⓒ Ⓓ
8. Ⓐ Ⓑ Ⓒ Ⓓ
9. Ⓐ Ⓑ Ⓒ Ⓓ

10. Ⓐ Ⓑ Ⓒ Ⓓ
11. Ⓐ Ⓑ Ⓒ Ⓓ
12. Ⓐ Ⓑ Ⓒ Ⓓ
13. Ⓐ Ⓑ Ⓒ Ⓓ
14. Ⓐ Ⓑ Ⓒ Ⓓ
15. Ⓐ Ⓑ Ⓒ Ⓓ
16. Ⓐ Ⓑ Ⓒ Ⓓ
17. Ⓐ Ⓑ Ⓒ Ⓓ
18. Ⓐ Ⓑ Ⓒ Ⓓ

19. Ⓐ Ⓑ Ⓒ Ⓓ
20. Ⓐ Ⓑ Ⓒ Ⓓ
21. Ⓐ Ⓑ Ⓒ Ⓓ
22. Ⓐ Ⓑ Ⓒ Ⓓ
23. Ⓐ Ⓑ Ⓒ Ⓓ
24. Ⓐ Ⓑ Ⓒ Ⓓ
25. Ⓐ Ⓑ Ⓒ Ⓓ
26. Ⓐ Ⓑ Ⓒ Ⓓ
27. Ⓐ Ⓑ Ⓒ Ⓓ

28. Ⓐ Ⓑ Ⓒ Ⓓ
29. Ⓐ Ⓑ Ⓒ Ⓓ
30. Ⓐ Ⓑ Ⓒ Ⓓ
31. Ⓐ Ⓑ Ⓒ Ⓓ
32. Ⓐ Ⓑ Ⓒ Ⓓ
33. Ⓐ Ⓑ Ⓒ Ⓓ
34. Ⓐ Ⓑ Ⓒ Ⓓ

Part 1: Reading

Time: 58 minutes

48 questions

QUESTIONS 1 THROUGH 6 ARE BASED ON THE FOLLOWING PASSAGE.

From *The Guilded Age*, by Mark Twain

"Even you and I will see the day that steamboats will come up that little Turkey river to within twenty miles of this land of ours—and in high water they'll come right to it! And this is not all, Nancy—it isn't even half! There's a bigger wonder—the railroad! These worms here have never even heard of it—and when they do they'll not believe in it. But it's another fact. Coaches that fly over the ground twenty miles an hour—heavens and earth, think of that, Nancy! Twenty miles an hour. It makes a man's brain whirl. Some day, when you and I are in our graves, there'll be a railroad stretching hundreds of miles—all the way down from the cities of the Northern States to New Orleans—and it's got to run within thirty miles of this land—may be even touch a corner of it.

…Pine forests, wheat land, corn land, iron, copper, coal—wait till the railroads come, and the steamboats! We'll never see the day, Nancy—never in the world—never, never, never, child. We've got to drag along, drag along, and eat crusts in toil and poverty, all hopeless and forlorn—but they'll ride in coaches, Nancy! They'll live like the princes of the earth; they'll be courted and worshiped; their names will be known from ocean to ocean! Ah, well-a-day! Will they ever come back here, on the railroad and the steamboat, and say, 'This one little spot shall not be touched—this hovel shall be sacred—for here our father and our mother suffered for us, thought for us, laid the foundations of our future as solid as the hills!'"

1. Which quotation is most representative of the title "The Guilded Age"?

    (A) "mother suffered for us"
    (B) "Even you and I will see the day"
    (C) "This one little spot shall not be touched"
    (D) "There's mountains of iron ore here"

2. If the reader continued to read this book what type of writing would be expected?

    (A) expository
    (B) narrative
    (C) persuasive
    (D) technical

3. What message was conveyed in the passage?

   (A) Things are better if left alone.
   (B) Progress is inevitable.
   (C) Chimneys should be built with care.
   (D) Change will not occur in the wilderness.

4. Which phrase is an expression of a stereotype in this passage?

   (A) "these worms here have never even heard of it"
   (B) "there'll be a railroad stretching hundreds of miles"
   (C) "eat crusts in toil and poverty"
   (D) "this hovel shall be sacred"

5. What is the author's position on the future based on this passage?

   (A) It will never be experienced.
   (B) It will be wonderful.
   (C) It will use up all resources.
   (D) It was thought of by their grandparents.

6. "These worms here have never even heard of it—and when they do they'll not believe in it." What is the meaning of *worms* in the above statement?

   (A) People to be respected.
   (B) People living close to the narrator.
   (C) People of low social status.
   (D) People of the future.

QUESTIONS 7 THROUGH 11 ARE BASED ON THE FOLLOWING PASSAGE.

Choose a colored pencil slightly lighter than the marker used for the garment for sheer fabric such as chiffon, tulle, organza, or crepe.

Color lightly in long, fluid, vertical lines beginning outside of the marker edge from left to right, ending outside of the marker edge on the right.

The more voluminous the fabric, the more colored pencil will be outside of the marker edge.

If the fabric has multiple tones or layers of color, repeat the colored pencil application on top of the previous layer, becoming lighter in color as you layer color.

Make an additional thick line of shadow on the left side, one-eighth inch from your other shadow line to draw silk, satin, or shiny fabric. The darker the shadow lines, the shinier the fabric will look.

Make the existing highlight line very light and thick. Make another thin highlight line, on the right side, about one-eighth inch from your other highlight. The lighter the highlights, the shinier the fabric will look.

Simplify a printed fabric into basic shapes and colors. Draw the print on top of the fabric with colored pencils. If you have a plaid or stripe, make a series of vertical stripes following the shape of the garment. Make the horizontal lines following the hem shape of the garment.

7. What would be the most likely title of the above passage?

   (A) Isn't color fun?
   (B) Your choices in color can be exciting!
   (C) How to color a clothing design drawing
   (D) What makes color vivid

8. This web page could be compared to which type of writing style?

   (A) expository
   (B) narrative
   (C) persuasive
   (D) technical

9. Choose rationale for identifying this passage as a secondary source of information.

   (A) This must be the only information source.
   (B) It was written after a theory was tested.
   (C) It seems to be a historical exposition.
   (D) The passage was based on a primary source.

10. What is the author's intended structure of this passage?

    (A) sequence
    (B) cause and effect
    (C) comparison and contrast
    (D) description

11. "The more voluminous the fabric, the more colored pencil will be outside of the marker edge." Which term best describes the information in this quote?

    (A) topic
    (B) supporting detail
    (C) main idea
    (D) theme

How can you catch a cold by not washing your hands? Germs may live on inanimate objects for an extended time. If you touch contaminated surfaces, the germs get on your hands. Eventually, you touch your eyes, nose, or mouth, which gives germs access to your insides.

12. Based on the above passage, what is the author's overall conclusion about hand washing?

    (A) Not washing your hands leads to more colds.
    (B) Inanimate objects cause colds.
    (C) The activity is not worth the effort.
    (D) Germs do not travel from objects to your insides.

With storm season around the corner and winter weather creeping in, it's the perfect time to put together your emergency kit. Your kit should include important items that you will need in an emergency, and a go bag of things you will need if you have to evacuate. Trying to get supplies after an emergency can be difficult. Roads may not be accessible, grocery stores may be closed, and other people may have also rushed out for supplies, emptying out the store shelves of what you need most.

13. Where would you most likely find the above passage?

    (A) first aid textbook

    (B) corporate newsletter

    (C) e-mail message from workplace

    (D) travel magazine

Nobody knows when a disaster might strike, but being prepared beforehand can help you survive. Whether it is a natural disaster in your local area, such as an earthquake or hurricane, or a man-made disaster, such as a terrorist attack or fire, you need to have survival kits and the proper emergency supplies. Disasters can force you to evacuate your neighborhood, workplace, or school, or they can confine you to your home. Having the right survival kits, first-aid kits, and emergency supplies on hand ahead of time is like having a spare tire in the trunk of your car. You hope not to have a flat tire, but it's nice to know that a spare tire is there, ready for use, to keep you going. Emergency preparedness is essential in this day and age.

14. On what public information channel would you expect to hear the above message?

    (A) emergency service bulletin

    (B) television alert

    (C) weather service announcement

    (D) tire center advertisement

You can't improve what you don't measure. The measuring stick for finances is a personal balance sheet, which lists what an individual owns and owes. Commit to updating your balance sheet every month. It takes just a few minutes, and this habit will cause you to refocus every month on your financial progress. In the words of Aristotle, "We are what we repeatedly do. Excellence, then, is not an act, but a habit." The same is true for financial freedom.

15. What is the overall message to the reader about financial stability in the above passage?

    (A) It is impossible.

    (B) It is a matter of repeating bad habits.

    (C) It can happen without any changes in behavior.

    (D) A personal balance sheet helps to refocus.

Why should sharks be saved? Sharks keep other prey species from becoming overabundant. Sharks keep the ocean clean by scavenging on dead animals. Sharks keep other species more fit by weeding out sick and weaker individuals. And sharks are beautiful, like lions and gorillas: crowning achievements of evolution.

16. What should the reader learn from the above article?

   (A) The killing of sharks is necessary.
   (B) Sharks do not have to be feared.
   (C) Sharks, like other animals, can be beneficial.
   (D) Watching sharks is dangerous.

The leader of the congregation of visitors from Europe expressed the idea of a tour of bird species around the world. The group was seeking rare birds and wanted to study some of the endangered species. Unfortunately the group would not be able to fulfill its goal since so many birds met the criteria for exploration and observation. The group split and decided to capture the birds on film. They reconvened to share their travels and all felt satisfaction with the results. They affirmed that the world is a great bird sanctuary and should be conserved. What a wonderful experience for all!

17. What type of manuscript is the above passage?

   (A) narrative
   (B) scientific essay
   (C) parody
   (D) short story

When an odorant stimulates the chemoreceptors in the nose that detect smell, they pass on electrical impulses to the brain. The brain then interprets patterns in electrical activity as specific odors and olfactory sensations become perception—something we recognize as smell. The only other chemical system that can as quickly identify, make sense of, and memorize new molecules is the immune system.

18. Which type of literature is the above passage most likely from?

   (A) textbook
   (B) science fiction novel
   (C) research journal
   (D) mystery novel

Jake wakes up to face the alien-acquired world 300 years from now and ends up being the only human survivor of the nuclear holocaust. All he has is a past life as an FBI agent, a few human clones around, and a big mission of saving the Earth and its resources from alien domination.

19. Which type of literature is the above passage most likely from?

   (A) textbook
   (B) science fiction novel
   (C) research journal
   (D) mystery novel

Member,

Earlier this week the House and Senate released a bipartisan FY 2014 Omnibus spending package that totaled $1.1 trillion. "This agreement shows the American people that we can compromise and that we can govern," Senate Appropriations Chairwoman, Barbara A. Mikulski (D-MD), said in a statement. "It puts an end to shutdown, slowdown, slam-down politics."

Thank you,

We are working for you in Washington!

20. What is the main purpose of the above e-mail?

   (A) The author wants to inform the reader.
   (B) The author wants to raise money for a cause.
   (C) The author disagrees with the way government operates.
   (D) The author wants to chat about basketball.

21. What is the author's bias regarding the theme mentioned in the e-mail?

   (A) Political action is always positive.
   (B) It is difficult to identify the author's bias.
   (C) He believes that spending controls are a great idea.
   (D) There are no biases noted.

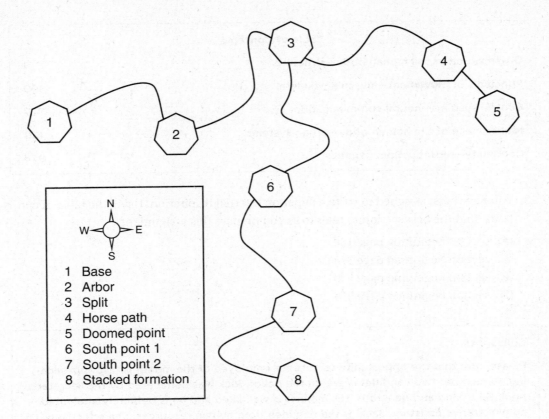

22. Based on the compass and key in the above figure, determine your location after following these directions.

Step 1. Depart from point 3.
Step 2. Travel south to the last point.
Step 3. Travel north three points.
Step 4. Travel east to next check point.
Where are you?

(A) base
(B) arbor
(C) horse path
(D) south point 1

Table of Contents	
Organization of the human body—structure	1
Principals of movement—muscular, skeletal	160
Control systems—neural communication	327
Maintenance of the human body—organ systems	610
Continuity—reproduction, genetics	974

23. You have been assigned to write a paper on internal respiration. Using the table of contents, find the best section to refer to as you prepare this assignment.

(A) section beginning page 160
(B) section beginning page 378
(C) section beginning page 610
(D) section beginning page 974

Colleagues,

Please note that the opportunity to vote for employee of the month is fast approaching. Remember two candidates are on the ballot. Rick was nominated by the secretarial pool. He is kind and generous. His manner is well liked and he is definitely a talented administrative assistant. Jacki is the nominee from human resources. She effectively provides personnel when needed for all departments. Her efficiency is evident every payday when we receive our checks.

Please vote for your choice by accessing the ballots online.

Thank you,

Sarah, Chair of Employee Rewards Committee

---

24. What is the author's bias in the above e-mail?

(A) Rick is the best candidate.
(B) It is difficult to identify the author's bias.
(C) Jacki is the best candidate.
(D) There are no biases noted.

25. The guide words at the top of a dictionary page are *litigious* and *loquacious*. Which word below could be located on this page?

(A) location
(B) liquation
(C) lux
(D) loma

26. A diner wants to order from the restaurant menu but needs to avoid chocolate and cow milk products. What should the person order?

   (A) cheeseburger macaroni casserole
   (B) salmon and gouda soufflé
   (C) strawberry yogurt parfait
   (D) chicken vegetable casserole

27. A traveler wants to visit the most famous historical site in Israel. Where would this traveler obtain the best information about the upcoming trip?

   (A) official guide to tourism in Israel
   (B) a recent documentary on travel in the Middle East
   (C) *International Travel News Journal*
   (D) *The Kosher Journal*

28. Edgar developed **ostentatious** habits after his promotion to president of the corporate branch. What is the definition of the word *ostentatious*?

   (A) bad taste or showy
   (B) appearance of unwarranted importance
   (C) vain display of opulence
   (D) expensive

29. Read the following directions.

   You are in charge of arranging items according to color and in pairs in the department store display. The display had one pair of each color: brown, black, white, green, red, and blue. After a sale the display has been depleted because the customers removed items, often only one item of a pair. You have added two blue items that were left over from the latest shipment. The customers removed one blue item, one red item, one white item, and two black items.

   How many pairs of same color items are now remaining?

   (A) 2
   (B) 3
   (C) 4
   (D) 6

PRODUCT	AMOUNT PER CONTAINER	AMOUNT ACTIVE INGREDIENT	PRICE	SPECIAL OFFER
Today O3	100	180 EPA	$4.95	4 for $19.30
YesOmega	500	180 EPA	$16.49	None
Omega Plus	60	50 EPA	$28.99	2 for $46.98
JustFish oil	100	Not stated	$7.19	5 for $23.98

30. You are planning to take fish oil to improve your heart and brain function.

    Which of the products in the above table would contain the highest active ingredient at the best price?

    (A) Today O3
    (B) YesOmega
    (C) Omega Plus
    (D) JustFish oil

QUESTIONS 31 AND 32 ARE BASED ON THE FOLLOWING PASSAGE.

The First-Lady Senator

Hillary Clinton was the oldest of three children born to Hugh and Dorothy Rodham. She grew up in Illinois and attended Wellesley College. After graduating in 1969, she attended Yale Law School. She practiced law in Little Rock, while working on behalf of children as Arkansas First Lady. Since becoming First Lady in 1993, she has continued her work in children's issues and human rights. She was the first female U.S. senator from New York State and won her first political office while still being First Lady.

31. Which choice best describes the title of the above passage?

    (A) topic
    (B) supporting detail
    (C) main idea
    (D) theme

32. What is the author's purpose in the above text?

    (A) to entertain
    (B) to persuade
    (C) to inform
    (D) to express feelings

33. The judge felt the punishment to be **capricious**. What is the meaning of *capricious*?

    (A) harsh
    (B) indecisive
    (C) short
    (D) unreasonable

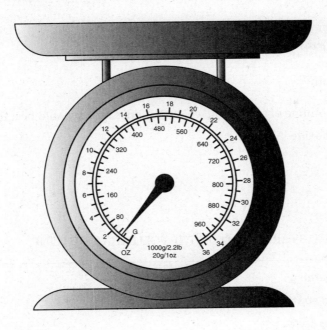

34. What is the maximum weight in grams that can be measured on the above scale?

    (A) 36
    (B) 72
    (C) 360
    (D) 1000

35. According to the weight on the above scale, how much will a product cost if it is priced at $32 per pound?

    (A) $0.20
    (B) $0.40
    (C) $2.00
    (D) $4.00

36. A supporter of a community leader running for chairman of the board wants to encourage others in the community to support his candidate. He decides to publish a letter. What department of the newspaper should be contacted?

    (A) editorial
    (B) business
    (C) classified
    (D) local news

37. Chapter 4: Electrolytes and Body Fluid

    (A) Sodium
    (B) Potassium
    (C) _____
    (D) Phosphate
    (E) Magnesium

    Based on the outline of Chapter 4, which response below would best fill in the blank?

    (A) Carbon dioxide
    (B) Calcium
    (C) Renin
    (D) Lactase

QUESTIONS 38 AND 39 ARE BASED ON THE FOLLOWING OUTLINE.

1. **Everyday Learning**

    A   Reading strategies

    B   Learning styles

    C   How to remember facts

2. **During the Test**

    A   Dealing with anxiety

    B   Test-taking strategies for multiple choice tests

    C   Test-taking strategies for essay tests

3. **After the Test**

    A   Tips to improve your scores in the next test

    B   Learning from your patterns

38. Identify the major section dealing with an after-exam review.

    (A) Everyday Learning
    (B) How to remember facts
    (C) Dealing with anxiety
    (D) Learning from your patterns

39. Identify the minor section that explains how to learn essential concepts based on your individual preferences.

    (A) Everyday Learning
    (B) Learning style
    (C) Test-taking strategies for multiple choice tests
    (D) Tips to improve your scores in the next test

	WINDOWS 7 ULTIMATE (64-BIT)	WINDOWS 8 (64-BIT)
Startup (seconds)	38	17
Shutdown (seconds)	12.2	9.9
500 MB File Group Move (seconds)	25.2	29.2
Large Single File Move (seconds)	46.4	46.8

40. A student is complaining that her computer is slower with Windows 8. According to the above table, which function in Windows 8 takes the longest?

    (A) Startup
    (B) Shutdown
    (C) 500 MB File Group Move
    (D) Large Single File Move

41. According to the above table, which function in Windows 7 is the slowest?

    (A) Startup
    (B) Shutdown
    (C) 500 MB File Group Move
    (D) Large Single File Move

QUESTIONS 42 AND 43 ARE BASED ON THE FOLLOWING LETTER.

Customer,

Please register online to pay your bill. It is convenient. You will not need to "worry" about late or incomplete payments again. Late fees will not apply. Your credit score will remain stable or improve.

Sign up today with Paybill or directly through bank withdrawal.

Thank you.

---

42. What is the message for the reader in this passage?

    (A) register
    (B) withdraw
    (C) sign up
    (D) worry

43. What is the meaning of the quotation marks in the passage?

    (A) to denote the beginning and end of a statement
    (B) to draw attention to the passage
    (C) to identify an opinion
    (D) to add emphasis to the word

44. In which section of the community guide would you find an acupuncturist?

(A) Auto Service
(B) Child Care
(C) Employment
(D) Health and Wellness

Food Cost Comparison

	JANUARY 1913	JANUARY 2013
Bread	$0.056	$1.422
Flour	$0.033	$0.524
Fresh milk, per gallon	$0.089/quart (or 0.356/gallon)	$3.526
Cheese	$0.222	$5.832
Butter	$0.409	$3.501
Coffee	$0.299	$5.902
Potatoes	$0.016	$0.627
Rice	$0.086	$0.715
Sirloin steak	$0.238	$5.705
Round steak	$0.205	$5.074
Chuck roast	$0.149	$3.696
Pork chops	$0.187	$3.465
Bacon	$0.254	$4.407
Ham	$0.251	$2.693
Eggs, per dozen	$0.373	$1.933
Sugar	$0.058	$0.683

45. Based on the above table, which food item has remained the most stable in cost since 1913?

(A) cheese
(B) flour
(C) milk
(D) sirloin steak

QUESTIONS 46 AND 47 ARE BASED ON THE FOLLOWING PASSAGE.

California is nearly as dry as it's ever been. High water marks rim half-full reservoirs. Cities are rationing water. Clerics are praying for rain. Ranchers are selling cattle, and farmers are fallowing fields.

46. Where is the reader likely to find the above passage?

(A) "People in the News" section
(B) science journal
(C) research article
(D) expressive writing newsletter

47. What is the meaning of *fallowing* in the above passage?

(A) to stay behind
(B) to foster change
(C) to plant small amounts
(D) to keep devoid of planting

48. Begin with the word *FIRST*. Follow the directions to make a new word.

Step 1. Move ST to the front of the word.
Step 2. Change the F to O.
Step 3. Remove I.
Step 4. Add E to the end of the word.

(A) stir
(B) stiff
(C) store
(D) strike

Part 2: Mathematics

Time: 51 minutes

34 questions

1. Simplify the expression: $(12 \div 4) \times 3 + 5 + 3 \times 5 - 2$.

    (A) 12
    (B) 27
    (C) 13
    (D) 23

2. Simplify the expression: $3 \times 6 \div 2 \times 3$.

    (A) 2
    (B) 7
    (C) 5
    (D) 3

3. Subtract 89,649 from 564,321.

    (A) 474,672
    (B) 746,724
    (C) 332,769
    (D) 624,650

4. Take 0.2163289 from 0.49463.

    (A) 1.2780
    (B) 278301
    (C) 0.2783
    (D) 2.7830

5. A student at the bookstore bought six $1.29 pens, two $0.99 erasers, and one $5.25 writing pad. How much did the student pay before tax?

    (A) $12.13
    (B) $8.52
    (C) $25.56
    (D) $14.97

6. A nurse is to give a 400-mg dose of a solution; the available vial has a strength of 500 mg in 20 milliliters. How many milliliters of this solution will the nurse give?

  (A) 20
  (B) 16
  (C) 10
  (D) 14

7. Compute the difference of $\frac{5}{4}-\frac{7}{12}$.

  (A) $1\frac{1}{2}$
  (B) $\frac{1}{3}$
  (C) $\frac{2}{3}$
  (D) $\frac{1}{2}$

8. What is the product of $0.25\times\frac{2}{7}$?

  (A) 0.0714
  (B) 1.0417
  (C) 0.1250
  (D) 0.2857

9. Divide 5 into $\frac{8}{3}$.

  (A) 0.33
  (B) 1.87
  (C) 2.67
  (D) 3.43

10. What irrational number is equivalent to the decimal 5.099?

  (A) square root of 23
  (B) square root of 18
  (C) square root of 31
  (D) square root of 26

11. Enrollment at a school goes from 850 to 910. What is the percent increase?

  (A) 12
  (B) 6
  (C) 7
  (D) 9

12. What is 43.5% in decimal form?

  (A) 0.435
  (B) 4.35
  (C) 43.5
  (D) 4/35

13. Which fraction is greater?

 (A) $\dfrac{3}{5}$

 (B) $\dfrac{2}{3}$

 (C) $\dfrac{6}{5}$

 (D) $\dfrac{5}{6}$

14. Estimate the sum of 46,951 + 34,947.

 (A) 71,898
 (B) 81,898
 (C) 79,986
 (D) 85,128

15. Reconcile this checking account for the current month. The previous balance was $2,564.93. Deposits were made for $125.47, $263.14, and $51.19; checks were written for $124.23, $65.60, and $75.15; and there is a service charge of $7. What is the balance?

 (A) $2,669.93
 (B) $2,639.75
 (C) $3,169.72
 (D) $2,732.75

16. An employee gets paid every other week. He works four 10-hour days per week and earns $22.50 per hour. Deductions include tax $255.92, retirement $75.50, and insurance $115.15. What is the take-home pay every other week?

 (A) $1,651.87
 (B) $1,442.52
 (C) $1,353.43
 (D) $1,553.35

17. A company's annual budget includes the following: salaries $350,500.50, supplies and ads $15,445.50, utilities $12,500.31, space lease $50,625.49, travel $25,425.82. What are the total expenses for the annual budget of this company?

 (A) $454,497.62
 (B) $544,253.62
 (C) $359,425.25
 (D) $625,463.49

18. A gathering is planned that expects an attendance of 42 people: 15 men and 27 women. The catering company charges $2.25 per lapel pin, $3.70 per flower corsage, $1.75 per cold drink, and $4 per cake serving. Men will get lapel pins, women will get flower corsages, and all will be served a cold drink and a piece of cake. What is the total cost?

 (A) $425.19
 (B) $375.15
 (C) $574.27
 (D) $421.19

19. A farmer made a feed mix consisting of the following components: 0.165 cooked rice, 0.036 hemp, and 0.137 crackers in a base of oatmeal. How much oatmeal is in the mix?

(A) 0.804
(B) 0.721
(C) 0.662
(D) 0.597

20. A realtor collects 7.2% of the selling price of each home sold. The realtor collected $21,210 in the last home sale. What was the selling price of the home?

(A) $495,382.25
(B) $385,246.73
(C) $223,985.77
(D) $294,583.33

21. A serving stand at a running event has the following fluids to distribute to 45 runners: 69 pints of water, 58 pints of lemonade, and 53 pints of electrolyte drinks. How many total pints of these beverages will be needed to distribute among 67 runners?

(A) 286
(B) 368
(C) 268
(D) 380

22. A medieval history book dates the "spread of the Black Death through Italy" in MCCCXLVIII. What is this date in conventional numbers?

(A) 1348
(B) 1358
(C) 1463
(D) 1238

23. A history record states that "Spain lost its 'invincible' armada in 1588." What is this date in Roman numerals?

(A) XVLXXXVIII
(B) MDLXXXVIII
(C) MDXXCVIII
(D) MVDLXXXVII

24. How many teaspoons are in 25 milliliters?

(A) 10
(B) 5
(C) 3
(D) 7

25. A gardener is to prepare 9 yards of soil for the next season. How many feet are in 9 yards?

   (A) 24
   (B) 18
   (C) 15
   (D) 27

26. A student needs to measure material for a device that will average 6.5 inches in width and $11\frac{3}{8}$ inches in length. What measurement tool is best to use in this case?

   (A) tape measure
   (B) meter stick
   (C) ruler
   (D) yardstick

27. On a blueprint of a robotic mechanism, 1 inch equals 24 inches. If the dimensions for the mechanism for height, width, and depth are 4 inches × 2 inches × 1 inch, respectively, what are the actual dimensions of the final product?

   (A) 24 × 9 × 3 feet
   (B) 8 × 4 × 2 feet
   (C) 12 × 6 × 3 feet
   (D) 9 × 4 × 3 feet

28. In Vince Lombardi's statement, "Perfection is not attainable, but if we chase perfection we can catch excellence," what is the independent variable?

   (A) perfection
   (B) chase
   (C) catch
   (D) excellence

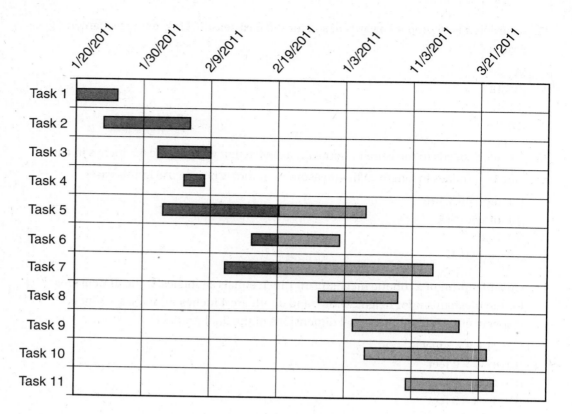

29. Based on the Gantt chart above, which tasks would take the longest to complete?

    (A) Tasks 1 and 2
    (B) Tasks 3 and 6
    (C) Tasks 5 and 7
    (D) Tasks 4 and 11

30. Of the following graph types, which would best represent a distribution around a mean?

    (A) Gantt
    (B) pie
    (C) line
    (D) histogram

31. Simplify the expression: $(12x^2 + 6xy - 3xy^2) \div (3xy)$.

    (A) $6x - 3 + y$
    (B) $4x + 2 - y$
    (C) $3(4x - 2y)$
    (D) $12x - 6y + 3$

32. Express the following into a mathematical expression: Matt is five times the age of his son Paul's age minus 7 years; if Paul's age is p, what is Matt's age?

    (A) $5(p+7)=x$

    (B) $7p-3=x$

    (C) $5p-7=x$

    (D) $-3+p=x$

33. Solve this equation for t: $t+8=15$.

    (A) 14

    (B) 3

    (C) 5

    (D) 7

34. Simplify the inequality: $|5x + 20| > 15$.

    (A) $x<7$ and $x>1$

    (B) $x<1$ and $x<7$

    (C) $x<1$ or $x>7$

    (D) $x<5$ or $x>35$

Part 3: Science

Time: 66 minutes

54 questions

QUESTIONS 1 AND 2 ARE BASED ON THE PERIODIC TABLE.

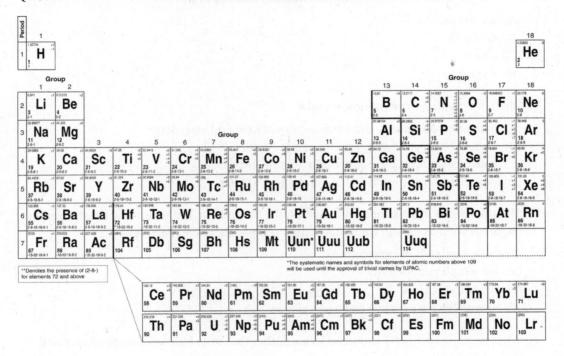

1. How many protons does sodium (NA) have?

   (A) 4
   (B) 8
   (C) 11
   (D) 16

2. How many neutrons does an atom of zinc (Zn) contain? The mass number is 65.39.

   (A) 12
   (B) 24
   (C) 28
   (D) 35

3. Which electromagnetic wave has the shortest wavelength?

   (A) green
   (B) infrared
   (C) X-rays
   (D) radio waves

4. A person pushes a cart a distance of 150 meters with a force of 50 N. What is the work done by the body?

   (A) 1,500 joules
   (B) 6,250 joules
   (C) 7,500 joules
   (D) 98,000 joules

5. What is the place on an enzyme that attaches to a substrate?

   (A) coenzyme
   (B) active site
   (C) catalyst
   (D) substrate

6. What are the properties of non-metals?

   (A) gain electrons easily, good conductors of heat and electricity
   (B) donate electrons easily, poor heat conductors
   (C) gain electrons easily, poor conductors of electricity
   (D) donate electrons easily, good conductors of heat

7. The transitions metals, located in the middle flat section of the periodic chart, contain elements such as Ag and Cn. What is their unique chemical reactivity?

   (A) have no free flowing electrons
   (B) have high conductivity
   (C) have drab colors
   (D) always have a negative electron valence

8. What chemical property is unique to a solution that tests blue with litmus paper and has a pH of 12?

   (A) will partially dissociate in a solution
   (B) has unstable cation
   (C) properties close to water
   (D) complete dissociation in solution

9. Which molecule found on Earth can also be found on other planets in the solar system?

   (A) oxygen
   (B) carbon dioxide
   (C) methane
   (D) propane

10. In order for covalent bonding to occur, what needs to be present?

    (A) Similar attractions of electrons between elements need to be present.
    (B) The elements will need to be to the left of the periodic chart.
    (C) The atoms must be on the same side of the periodic chart.
    (D) Dissimilar electronegativity needs to be present.

11. How many molecules of H_2O will be needed to balance this equation?
    $$\_\_ \text{ KOH} + \_\_ \text{ H}_3\text{PO}_4 \rightarrow \_\_ \text{ K}_3\text{PO}_4 + \_\_ \text{ H}_2\text{O}$$

    (A) 1
    (B) 2
    (C) 3
    (D) 5

12. Why doesn't a glass full of ice and water overflow if the ice melts?

    (A) The density of water changes when frozen.
    (B) The ice continues to float on top.
    (C) The water evaporates as ice melts.
    (D) The capillary action would hold the water in place.

13. What is an example of a gas that moves directly from a solid to the gaseous state without additional heat?

    (A) oxygen
    (B) carbon dioxide
    (C) carbon monoxide
    (D) chlorine

14. Which hypothesis is testable and meets scientific rigor for hypothesis testing?

    (A) There is a relationship between type of surgery and resulting pain levels after the procedure.
    (B) People who drink tea are happy.
    (C) Dogs are more fun after behavior training.
    (D) The goal is to discover the best brand of hydrogen peroxide to use on a cut.

15. Which of these statements would suggest that a directional hypothesis was formulated?

    (A) Children will be followed over time to determine the effect of online tutorials on science scores.
    (B) There will be no difference in the SAT scores of home schooled children who completed online chemistry quizzes and the public school student's scores.
    (C) There was a question whether a home schooled child could learn chemistry online.
    (D) Children can learn topics online.

16. A research team has discovered that a substance that they had been researching has some undesirable characteristics and they are considering what to do now. In what phase of the scientific process are they currently working?

    (A) problem identification
    (B) question asking
    (C) data collection
    (D) experimenting

17. This research team is trying to find out if there is commonality of thought about a certain phenomenon and seek to collect information online. Which of these designs would fit?

    (A) non-experimental design
    (B) qualitative design
    (C) experimental design
    (D) survey

18. Which research variable(s) would be the main outcome of interest?

    (A) independent
    (B) dependent
    (C) both independent and dependent
    (D) neither independent nor dependent

19. In a study called "How does pain affect sleep?" what are the dependent and independent variables?

    (A) does, affect
    (B) pain, sleep
    (C) how, sleep
    (D) sleep, pain

20. There is a newly discovered herbal medication. The team wants to find out why people would even take the substance. There is very little data. What type of study design is this?

    (A) either qualitative or quantitative
    (B) quantitative
    (C) qualitative
    (D) mixed

21. The researcher has found that there is an established theory on sedentary lifestyle but wants to make sure it applies to people who live in China. What type of reasoning would apply to this study?

    (A) quantitative
    (B) deductive
    (C) inductive
    (D) proactive

22. The research team is planning to collect data on a phenomenon after an intervention with a pre-test and post-test instrument. Which of these designs would fit?

   (A) non-experimental design
   (B) qualitative design
   (C) experimental design
   (D) survey

23. How should a researcher test the research question that suggests that eating apples reduces heartburn?

   (A) Randomly divide study participants into groups, measure the severity of heartburn pain before providing apples or no fruit to the groups, and then measure severity of heartburn one hour after the food.
   (B) Have each randomly divided group of study participants consume the apples each day and follow up after one week.
   (C) Suggest apples and ask study participants to map their own relief from their heartburn.
   (D) Randomly divide study participants into groups, measure the severity of heart-burn pain before providing the apples to one group, provide a placebo to the other group, then measure severity of heartburn one hour after the food or placebo group were given apples or no fruit.

24. In the biological classification system families are grouped under which hierarchy?

   (A) orders
   (B) genus
   (C) species
   (D) divisions

25. In an adaptation environment why would animals develop blubber?

   (A) climate change
   (B) predators
   (C) availability of food
   (D) increased mating opportunities

26. Which of these is a nucleic acid?

   (A) amino acid
   (B) enzymes
   (C) lipase
   (D) RNA

27. Which cellular organelle removes cellular debris?

   (A) lysosomes
   (B) mitochondrion
   (C) Golgi apparatus
   (D) ribosomes

28. What happens to an individual that has an X and Y chromosome?

    (A) That person will be female.

    (B) That person will be male.

    (C) That person will have male and female genitalia.

    (D) The person will be extremely intelligent.

29. How many haploid cells result from meiosis?

    (A) two

    (B) four

    (C) eight

    (D) one

30. What structure would NOT be in a bacterial cell?

    (A) DNA

    (B) cell membrane

    (C) Golgi apparatus

    (D) ribosomes

31. If a tall plant is crossed with a short plant, what would be the expected outcome in Mendelian genetics?

    (A) all short

    (B) all tall

    (C) all medium

    (D) half tall, half short

32. What is the classical symptom of most infectious diseases?

    (A) fever

    (B) jaundice

    (C) vomiting

    (D) pain

33. Which is the antibody of a primary immune response?

    (A) IgG

    (B) IgM

    (C) IgA

    (D) IgE

34. A child has blue eyes (bb). The mother has blue eyes and the father has brown eyes. Which of these would represent the father in a genetic chart?

    (A) bb

    (B) Bb

    (C) BB

    (D) Bbb

35. What is the protein most important for DNA replication?

    (A) RNA polymerase
    (B) transfer RNA
    (C) messenger RNA
    (D) DNA polymerase

36. What is the function of the pericardium?

    (A) provide a barrier against infection
    (B) improve blood flow through the heart
    (C) help with cardiac conduction system
    (D) help with cardiac contraction

37. What would happen to the heart rate if a person took a medication that stimulated the sympathetic nervous system?

    (A) decreased strength of the ventricular contraction
    (B) decreased heart rate
    (C) increased heart rate
    (D) increased AV node conduction

38. Where does coronary venous blood drain into the heart?

    (A) superior vena cava
    (B) inferior vena cava
    (C) right atrium
    (D) left atrium

39. Which of the following structures is primarily responsible for sneezing?

    (A) upper respiratory tract mucosa
    (B) irritant receptors in the trachea and large airways
    (C) irritant receptors in the nostrils
    (D) nasal hairs and turbinates

40. What is the area of the brain most likely involved with respiration?

    (A) cerebral cortex
    (B) thalamus
    (C) basal ganglia
    (D) brain stem

41. What are receptors in the lung that decrease ventilatory rate and volume when stimulated?

    (A) carbon dioxide receptors
    (B) baroreceptors
    (C) stretch receptors
    (D) chemoreceptors

42. Keratinocytes are found in which layer of the skin?

    (A) epidermis
    (B) papillary layer of the dermis
    (C) reticular layer of the dermis
    (D) hypodermis

43. Which of these structures is contained within the nephron?

    (A) loop of Henle
    (B) urethra
    (C) renal capsule
    (D) renal pelvis

44. How is the renin-angiotensin system activated?

    (A) increased blood volume
    (B) elevated sodium concentrations
    (C) decreased blood pressure in the afferent arterioles
    (D) renal hypoxia

45. What role do the kidneys play in vitamin D function?

    (A) synthesizing vitamin D from cholesterol
    (B) activating intestinally absorbed vitamin D
    (C) metabolizing and breaking down vitamin D
    (D) excreting excess vitamin D

46. What is the transverse fiber tract that connects the two cerebral hemispheres?

    (A) peduncle
    (B) corpus callosum
    (C) basal ganglia
    (D) pons

47. What causes hydrocephalus?

    (A) blockage of cerebral aqueduct
    (B) blockage of inferior colliculi
    (C) blockage of red nucleus
    (D) blockage of tegmentum

48. Which is a sensory pathway of the spinal cord?

    (A) corticospinal tract
    (B) pyramids
    (C) spinothalamic tract
    (D) anterior column

49. What is the outermost membrane surrounding the brain?

    (A) dura mater
    (B) arachnoid mater
    (C) pia mater
    (D) falx cerebri

50. How much of the cardiac output does the brain receive?

    (A) 80%
    (B) 20%
    (C) 40%
    (D) 10%

51. What process regulates insulin?

    (A) metabolic rate
    (B) serum glucose levels
    (C) prostaglandins
    (D) enzyme activation

52. Which hormone is secreted by the adrenal medulla?

    (A) cortisol
    (B) epinephrine
    (C) androgens
    (D) estrogens

53. A blood sample is analyzed in a laboratory. Assuming a normal sample, which type of white blood cell accounts for the highest percentage?

    (A) neutrophils
    (B) eosinophils
    (C) monocytes
    (D) lymphocytes

54. What is the predominant phagocyte of early inflammation?

    (A) eosinophil
    (B) lymphocyte
    (C) macrophage
    (D) neutrophil

Part 4: English and Language Usage

Time: 34 minutes

34 questions

1. Lorna **longingly** anticipated her return home after the long stay in her faraway corporation.

   The word *longingly* serves as which part of speech in the sentence above?

   (A) verb
   (B) adjective
   (C) adverb
   (D) possessive

2. The <u>boys</u> who played <u>harder</u> tired first.
   Which of the following correctly identifies the parts of speech in the underlined portions of the sentence?

   (A) subject; adverb
   (B) subject; object
   (C) adjective; clause
   (D) article; clause

3. Which of the following sentences has correct subject–verb agreement?

   (A) John and Joni, the out-of-town twins, likes to sit in the upfront pews.
   (B) John and Joni, the out-of-town twins, like to sit in the upfront pews.
   (C) A clique of siblings who just moved into town like to sit in the upfront pews.
   (D) Most of the families who come to visit likes to sit in the upfront pews.

4. Which of the following sentences provides an example of correct subject–verb agreement?

   (A) When the plane begins to take off, every one of the passengers buckle up.
   (B) Since their flight was delayed, the crew of award winners arrive late to the reception.
   (C) When the eatery weekly offers free-dessert nights, the whole town seemingly shows up.
   (D) The team of twelve players arrive too early because the chronometer was ignored.

5. Facing sustained hardship, <u>Bob</u> was thrilled when Christine told ___ of the overwhelming demand for the product in the upcoming season.

Which of the following options is the correct pronoun for the sentence above? The antecedent of the pronoun to be added is underlined.

(A) it
(B) him
(C) them
(D) her

6. Alerted by the reliable rooster, the flock compliantly flew to __ safety in the hencoop. Which of the following is the correct pronoun to complete the sentence above?

(A) its
(B) their
(C) it's
(D) there

7. Which of the following is an example of a correctly punctuated direct dialogue sentence?

(A) In the tragedy play *Hamlet*, the king says, "O, speak of that; that do I long to hear."
(B) In the tragedy play *Hamlet*, the king "says, O, speak of that;" that do I "long to hear."
(C) In the tragedy play *Hamlet*, the king says, O, speak of that; that do I long to hear.
(D) In the tragedy play *Hamlet*, the king says, "O, speak of 'that'; that do I 'long' to hear."

8. Which of the following sentences correctly punctuates direct dialogue?

(A) In the allegory *The Pilgrim's Progress*, the protagonist acts thus, and not being able longer to contain, he brake out with a lamentable cry, saying—"What shall I do?"
(B) In the allegory *The Pilgrim's Progress*, the protagonist acts thus, "and not being able longer to contain, he brake out with a lamentable cry, saying—'What shall I do?'"
(C) In the allegory *The Pilgrim's Progress*, the protagonist acts thus, 'and not being able longer to contain,' he brake out with a lamentable cry, saying—'What shall I do?'
(D) In the allegory "The Pilgrim's Progress," the protagonist acts thus, "and not being able longer to contain, he brake out with a lamentable cry," saying—What shall I do?

9. Which of the following is an example of third-person point of view?

(A) We suggest for you to leave the event an hour before its end to avoid the evening traffic.
(B) Heidi and I wanted to leave the event an hour before its end to avoid the evening traffic.
(C) Gail and Gus chose to leave the event an hour before its end to avoid the heavy traffic.
(D) You have to decide to leave the event an hour before its end to avoid the heavy traffic.

10. Which of the following sentences in the instructions below is an example of first-person voice?

(A) As soon as you see the curve, make a right and then a quick left turn.
(B) Once anyone sees the curve, it is easy to make the right and quick left turns.
(C) As soon as I missed the curve, there was no way to turn right and then left.
(D) After they saw the curve, we failed to see the way to turn right and then left.

11. Tiff was studying for the exam. She stumbled on a new term. She searched the glossary. The word was not defined.

Which of the following options best uses grammar for style and clarity to combine the sentences above?

(A) Tiff was studying for the exam when she stumbled on a new term; when she searched the glossary, the word was not defined.
(B) Tiff stumbled on a new term as she studied for the exam, then the word was not defined when she searched the glossary.
(C) Tiff searched the glossary because she stumbled on a new term while studying for the exam, but the word was not defined.
(D) Tiff searched the glossary, she stumbled on a new term while she was studying for the exam, but the word was not defined.

12. Dave had a low fever. He felt well. His mom got worried. She called the doctor.

Which of the following options best uses grammar for style and clarity to combine the sentences above?

(A) Dave had low fever but felt well, his mom got worried and called the doctor.
(B) Although he felt well, Dave had low fever; his mom called the doctor because she got worried.
(C) His mom got worried because Dave had low fever though he felt well; so she called the doctor.
(D) Despite his low fever Dave felt well, but his mom got worried and called the doctor.

13. In his hopeless avarice, he could not help **coveting** funds.

Which of the following is the meaning of the word *coveting* as used in the sentence above?

(A) charity
(B) greed
(C) concealing
(D) payment

14. She tried to do a fair critique of the new horror story, but she could not hide her love for the **macabre**.

Which of the following is the meaning of the word *macabre*?

(A) amusing
(B) thrill
(C) ghoulish
(D) burlesque

15. Mike's condition has greatly improved; he attributes that to his phytonutrient supplement.

    In the sentence above, the prefix *phyto-* in *phytonutrient* indicates that the term is related to what?

    (A) intake of plant compounds
    (B) intake of synthetic blends
    (C) intake of animal products
    (D) intake of mineral mixtures

16. The new student dislikes arithmetic, and she claims to have a serious case of numerophobia.

    In the sentence above, the suffix *-phobia* in *numerophobia* can best be defined by which of the following words?

    (A) belief in
    (B) love for
    (C) fear of
    (D) study of

17. Which of the following words is spelled correctly?

    (A) greivous
    (B) awesome
    (C) trueism
    (D) gloryous

18. Which of the following words is spelled correctly?

    (A) exagerate
    (B) forfeit
    (C) grievose
    (D) hessitancy

19. He had chronic _____ and moving to the smoggy city was not to his advantage.

    Which of the following options correctly completes the sentence above?

    (A) bloating
    (B) depression
    (C) migraines
    (D) emphysema

20. When we went ___ town we bought ___ books; Wen ___ did so.

    Which of the following options correctly complete the question above?

    (A) too; to; two
    (B) to; two; too
    (C) two; too; to
    (D) too; to; two

21. The hurricane's destruction barely missed my area, I <u>scarsely</u> got away unhurt.

    Which of the following words corrects the spelling of the underlined word above?

    (A) scarcely
    (B) scarlesly
    (C) scarily
    (D) scaresly

22. Which of the underlined words is an example of correct spelling, considering the context of the sentence.

    (A) She said that the new ingredient would have no <u>affect</u> on the original product.
    (B) He based his overall decision on the <u>principal</u> of autonomy.
    (C) At the start of the adventure, they knew not where <u>they're</u> journey would end.
    (D) We'll start from separate points and then meet at the <u>ascent</u> of the hill.

23. Which of the following sentences follows the rules of capitalization?

    (A) H. Benjamin was a doctor who used diet to treat disease.
    (B) Tolstoy's War and peace is a monumental novel.
    (C) They said they would be here sunday afternoon.
    (D) We decided next time to travel through Eastern Tennessee.

24. When we go to England, we'd like to visit the British Museum with its many exhibits of ancient world artifacts, and also see panoramic countryside, such as the outstanding beauty of the cotswolds.

    Which of the following words in the sentence above should be capitalized?

    (A) ancient
    (B) world
    (C) panoramic
    (D) cotswolds

25. Which of the following sentences correctly applies the rules of punctuation?

    (A) She only talked to uninterested boys: if one showed any interest, she ignored him.
    (B) She only talked to uninterested boys; if one showed any interest, she ignored him.
    (C) She only talked to uninterested boys, if one showed any interest, she ignored him.
    (D) She only talked to uninterested boys, if one showed any interest, she ignored him.

26. The gourmet meal was tasteful, the dessert was addicting __I could not stop eating.
    Which of the following punctuation marks correctly completes the sentence above?

    (A) –
    (B) ,
    (C) ( )
    (D) .

27. Which of the following is an example of a simple sentence?

    (A) You and Jean alone followed the instructions correctly, so you did a great job.
    (B) Only you and Jean followed the instructions correctly and did a great job.
    (C) Because you and Jean followed the instructions correctly, you did a great job.
    (D) By following the instructions correctly the job done by you and Jean was great.

28. The computer technician with the ponytail and the baggy pants...

    Which of the following completions for the above sentence results in a simple sentence structure?

    (A) solves most glitches faster, so more consumers prefer him.
    (B) attracted most consumers because he consistently solved more glitches.
    (C) attracts most consumers lately, as their new glitches are quickly solved by him.
    (D) attracted more consumers and solved most of the glitches.

29. Mike admired the new car models. He was annoyed by the steep price tags.

    Which of the following uses a conjunction to combine the sentences above so that the focus is more on Mike's admiring the cars, and less on his being annoyed?

    (A) Mike admired the new car models; he was annoyed by the steep price tags.
    (B) Mike admired the new car models and was annoyed by the pricey tags.
    (C) Mike was annoyed by the pricey tags, but he admired the new car models.
    (D) Mike was annoyed by the pricey tags, though he admired the new car models.

30. The new economics graduate...

    Which of the following allows the above sentence to be completed as a simple sentence?

    (A) was warned to avoid risky ventures but liked aggressive transactions.
    (B) was warned to avoid risky ventures; nonetheless, she loved aggressive transactions.
    (C) liked aggressive transactions, although warned of avoiding risky ventures.
    (D) loved aggressive transactions, she was warned about risky ventures.

31. Which of the following sentences is most clear and correct?

    (A) She's ever beautiful, though after three decades of being in the limelight.
    (B) After three decades in the limelight she's ever beautiful.
    (C) In the limelight after three decades still she's ever beautiful.
    (D) Even after three decades in the limelight she's ever beautiful.

32. Kate's parent traveled abroad. She stayed home. She felt lonely. She called her friends. To improve sentence fluency, which of the following best states the information above in a single sentence?

    (A) When Kate's parents traveled abroad, she stayed home and felt lonely, so she called her friends.
    (B) While Kate's parents traveled abroad and she stayed home, she felt lonely and called her friends.
    (C) Kate's parents traveled abroad, she stayed home and felt lonely and called her friends.
    (D) When her parents traveled abroad, and Kate felt lonely as she stayed home, she called her friends.

33. Lou went fishing. The weather was right. The lake was quiet. He caught nothing.

To improve sentence fluency, which of the following best states the information above in a single sentence?

(A) Lou went fishing when the weather was right, the lake was quiet but he caught nothing.

(B) While the weather was right and the lake was quiet, Lou went fishing and caught nothing.

(C) Lou caught nothing though he went fishing when the weather was right and the lake was quiet.

(D) The weather was right when Lou went fishing, the lake was quiet yet he caught nothing.

34. We attended the meeting. The snacks were lousy. The agenda was dull. We absconded.

To improve sentence fluency, which of the following best states the information above in a single sentence?

(A) We attended the meeting, the snacks were lousy and the agenda was dull, we absconded.

(B) The snacks were lousy and the agenda was dull, so we absconded when we attended the meeting.

(C) When we attended the meeting the agenda was dull, we absconded (the snacks were lousy).

(D) We attended the meeting and absconded; besides, the agenda was dull and the snacks were lousy.

ANSWER KEY
Practice Test 5

READING

1.	B	13.	A	25.	A	37.	B
2.	B	14.	A	26.	D	38.	D
3.	B	15.	D	27.	A	39.	B
4.	A	16.	C	28.	C	40.	C
5.	B	17.	A	29.	B	41.	A
6.	B	18.	A	30.	B	42.	A
7.	C	19.	B	31.	C	43.	B
8.	D	20.	A	32.	C	44.	D
9.	D	21.	C	33.	D	45.	B
10.	A	22.	C	34.	D	46.	B
11.	B	23.	C	35.	C	47.	D
12.	A	24.	B	36.	A	48.	C

MATHEMATICS

1.	B	10.	D	19.	C	28.	A
2.	D	11.	C	20.	D	29.	C
3.	A	12.	A	21.	C	30.	D
4.	C	13.	C	22.	A	31.	B
5.	D	14.	B	23.	B	32.	C
6.	B	15.	D	24.	B	33.	D
7.	C	16.	C	25.	D	34.	C
8.	A	17.	A	26.	C		
9.	B	18.	B	27.	B		

SCIENCE

1. C	15. A	29. B	43. A
2. D	16. B	30. B	44. C
3. C	17. A	31. B	45. B
4. C	18. B	32. A	46. B
5. B	19. D	33. B	47. A
6. C	20. C	34. C	48. C
7. B	21. B	35. C	49. A
8. D	22. C	36. A	50. B
9. C	23. D	37. C	51. A
10. A	24. A	38. C	52. B
11. C	25. A	39. A	53. A
12. A	26. D	40. D	54. A
13. B	27. A	41. C	
14. A	28. B	42. A	

ENGLISH AND LANGUAGE USAGE

1. B	10. C	19. D	28. D
2. A	11. C	20. B	29. C
3. B	12. D	21. A	30. A
4. C	13. B	22. D	31. D
5. B	14. C	23. A	32. D
6. C	15. A	24. D	33. C
7. A	16. C	25. B	34. C
8. B	17. B	26. C	
9. C	18. B	27. B	

ANSWER EXPLANATIONS

Reading

1. **(B)** The quote that best represents the title of the work is "Even you and I will see the day." The title describes the time and effects of an expanding economy on everyone.

2. **(B)** Narrative style tells a story. Expository passages explain a topic or subject in order to increase understanding of ideas. Technical writing usually addresses precise information. Persuasive writing tries to convince the reader to agree with the author.

3. **(B)** This is the general idea expressed by the author. The other choices reflect more incorrect assumptions not expressed in the passage.

4. **(A)** A stereotype is a statement or opinion about an entire group of people. The other statements are negative but are not directed at individuals.

5. **(B)** The overall progression of the message is directed toward the wonder of the future. The other statements, although present in the passage, are supporting details that help support how awesome the future can be.

6. **(B)** This response best describes the narrators living close to the concerned location. None of the other answers are discussed in the work.

7. **(C)** This is an article on how to color a clothing design drawing.

8. **(D)** This example of technical writing expresses precise information on how to effectively present color in a fashion draft. Persuasive writing tries to convince the reader to agree with the author. Narrative style tells a story.

9. **(D)** This is a general information site so the passage would be based on another source.

10. **(A)** This is a sequence expressed as a list. A comparison–contrast structure has two opposing ideas that force the reader to identify a difference. The cause and effect structure would describe an event with expected consequences.

11. **(B)** This is a supporting detail. The topic or main idea is how to color a pattern or fashion diagram.

12. **(A)** The overall intent of the passage is to explain the relationship between washing your hands and getting a cold.

13. **(A)** The passage seems to be from a first aid textbook and is intended to give information. The author was not trying to persuade you to purchase something or trying to get you to laugh.

14. **(A)** The passage is from an emergency service bulletin.

15. **(D)** This article introduces the reader to the benefits of a personal balance sheet.

16. **(C)** The overall purpose is to reassure the reader that sharks have a purpose and should not be destroyed. The other answers are incorrect and reflect ideas that oppose that of the writer.

17. **(A)** This was written in a narrative style.

18. **(A)** This passage could be a sample from a science textbook.

19. **(B)** This is most likely taken from a novel since it was written to entertain. It hints at the supernatural so it is likely science fiction. It is not from a textbook since it is not purely informative in nature.

20. **(A)** The e-mail is definitely written to inform members of a service provided.

21. **(C)** It was openly written that the author is in favor of the Omnibus Spending Bill.

22. **(C)** Step 1. Depart from point 3. (Split)
Step 2. Travel south to the last point. (Stacked Formation)
Step 3. Travel north three points. (Split)
Step 4. Travel east to next check point. (Horse path)

23. **(C)** The lungs (an organ system) are in charge of respiration.

24. **(B)** The author has positives to say about both employees nominated for the award. It is difficult to identify the author's bias. There seems to be more written about one candidate than the other so D is incorrect.

25. **(A)** *Location* would be found on this page.

26. **(D)** The only dish listed without chocolate or milk products is chicken vegetable casserole. Cheese contains milk, gouda is a type of cheese, and yogurt is a milk product.

27. **(A)** A is the most reliable source. B and C responses are too general and D is a specific type of regional cooking.

28. **(C)** *Ostentatious* means a display of opulence with accompanying vanity. B is a better definition for *pretentious*.

29. **(B)** The customers have removed odd items from a white, red, blue, and black pair. That would leave only two remaining pairs. One blue pair was replaced. So there are only three complete pairs remaining.

30. **(B)** The YesOmega brand has the recommended dose of EPA at the best price: $0.03 per capsule. Today O3 is about $0.05, and Omega Plus and JustFish oil are not at the highest active ingredient level.

31. **(C)** Hillary Rodham Clinton is the topic. The fact that she was more than just a First Lady is the main idea.

32. **(C)** The author's intent is to inform the reader with facts about a historic person.

33. **(D)** *Capricious* is defined as "unreasonable, unpredictable."

34. **(D)** The highest measurement on this weight scale is 1000 grams or 36 ounces.

35. **(C)** There are 16 ounces in a pound. 32 divided by 16 = $2.00.

36. **(A)** This type of letter would be a letter to the editor of the local newspaper.

37. **(B)** Calcium is the only electrolyte in the answer list.

38. **(D)** This statement is located in "After your exam."

39. **(B)** Learning style assessments allow you to determine how you will learn most effectively.

40. **(C)** The only great difference in speed between the two systems is the 500 MB File Group Move.

41. **(A)** Startup in Windows 7 is twice as slow as in Windows 8.

42. **(A)** This is meant to persuade the reader to pay bills online.

43. **(B)** The quotation marks create emphasis to draw attention to the word *worry*.

44. **(D)** The community guide would list an acupuncturist under "Health and Wellness."

45. **(B)** Flour has only increased in cost $0.49.

46. **(B)** This would likely appear in a science journal.

47. **(D)** *Fallow* means that the fields are left plowed under without plants.

48. **(C)** Step 1. Move ST to the front of the word. (STFIR)
    Step 2. Change the F to O. (STOIR)
    Step 3. Remove I. (STOR)
    Step 4. Add an E to the end of the word. (STORE)

Mathematics

1. **(B)** $\left(\dfrac{12}{4}\right) \times 3 + 5 + 3 \times 5 - 2 = 3 \times 3 + 5 + 3 \times 5 - 2$

$$= 9 + 5 + 15 - 2$$
$$= 27$$

Simplify the expression with the innermost parentheses first, next multiply, then add and subtract.

2. **(D)** $-\dfrac{(3 \times 6)}{2 \times 3} = \dfrac{18}{6} = 3$

3. **(A)** 564321
    −89649
    474672

When subtracting whole numbers, numbers are arranged in columns with like place values in each column.

4. **(C)** This option is correct. Thus,

    0.49463000
    −0.42163289
    0.27830111 or 0.2783 .

5. **(D)** This is the only option; thus, six $1.29 pens, two $0.99 erasers, and one $5.25 writing pad works out as:

    (6 × $1.29) + (2 × $0.99) + $5.25 = $14.97.

6. **(B)** Since there are 500 milligrams in 20 milliliters, the nurse will give 16 milliliters for a strength of 400 milligrams. Cross-multiply: 500 mg/20 ml = 400 mg/x ml

$$500x = (400)(20)$$
$$x = \frac{8,000}{500}$$
$$x = 16 \text{ ml}$$

7. **(C)** Find the lowest common denominator. Then solve: $\dfrac{5}{4} - \dfrac{7}{12} = \dfrac{15}{12} - \dfrac{7}{12} = \dfrac{8}{12} = \dfrac{2}{3}$.

8. **(A)** $0.25 \times \dfrac{2}{7} = 0.25 \times 0.285714286 = 0.071428571$ or 0.0714

   Convert the fraction to a decimal to work with like numbers, then multiply.

9. **(B)** Convert the fraction to a decimal, and rewrite the given expression accordingly. So, $\dfrac{5}{2.67} = 1.87$.

10. **(D)** The decimal form 5.099 is greater than the square root of 25 and less than the square root of 16. Since options A and B are too small, and option C is too big, the only option left is D.

11. **(C)** $\dfrac{(910 - 850)}{850} = 7\%$ decrease.

12. **(A)** 43.5% converts to a decimal by removing the % sign and moving the decimal point two places left: 43.5% = 0.435.

13. **(C)** First find the common denominator; then the fraction with the greater numerator will be greater.

14. **(B)** Since this is an estimate, start by rounding all integers to easier numbers and compare. So, 4700 − 3500 = 8200. Because options A and C are too low and option D is too high, the only possible option is B.

15. **(D)** (2,564.93 + 125.47 + 263.14 + 51.19) − (124.23 + 65.60 + 75.15 + 7) = $2,732.75

16. **(C)** ($22.50 × 40 hours × 2 weeks = $1800 beginning salary) − (255.92 + 75.50 + 115.15 = $446.57 expenses) = $1353.43 take-home salary.

17. **(A)** All added expenses are: 350,500.50 + 15,445.50 + 12,500.31 + 50,625.49 + 25,425.82 = $454,497.62.

18. **(B)** (15 × $2.25 = $33.75) + (27 × $3.70 = $99.90) + (42 × $1.75 = $73.50) + (42 × $4 = $168) = $375.15

19. **(C)** 0.165 rice + 0.036 hemp + 0.137 crackers = 0.338. Then, 1.000 (whole mix) − 0.338 (three ingredients) = 0.662 oatmeal.

20. **(D)** 7.2% = 0.072 in decimal form. Convert the percent to a decimal and divide by the decimal obtained. Thus,

$$\frac{2121}{0.072} = \$294,583.33.$$

21. **(C)** 69 + 58 + 53 = 180 beverages for 45 runners. Cross-multiply to compute that amount for 67 runners. Thus,

$$\frac{67}{x} = \frac{45}{180} = \frac{12{,}060}{45}$$

$$x = \frac{12{,}060}{45}$$

$x = 268$ beverages.

22. **(A)** M = 1000, C = 100, L = 50, X = 10, V = 5, I = 1. If a smaller number is listed before M, L, X, or V, it will be subtracted from the main number. Traditionally, the numbers that follow in decreasing number add to the total number. Thus, M = 1000, CCC = 300 (100 × 3), XL = 40 (50 − 40), VIII = 8 (5 + 3).

23. **(B)** M = 1000, D = 500, C = 100, L = 50, X = 10, V = 5, I = 1. Traditionally, the numbers that follow in decreasing number add to the total number. Thus, M = 1000, D = 500, LXXX = 80 (50 + 30), VIII = 8 (5 + 3).

24. **(B)** 5 milliliters = 1 teaspoon. Thus, 25 milliliters = 5 teaspoons.

25. **(D)** 1 yard = 3 feet. Thus, 9 yards = 27 feet.

26. **(C)** In this case the materials being measured are all larger than 6 inches and smaller than 12 inches; therefore, a ruler would be most appropriate.

27. **(B)** 1 inch = 24 inches (2 feet). Then, the actual dimensions are (2 × 4), (2 × 2), and (2 × 1) = 8 feet × 4 feet × 2 feet.

28. **(A)** The independent variable is the input which is put into the set of data.

29. **(C)** Based on the Gantt chart, tasks 5 and 7 would take the longest time to complete.

30. **(D)** A histogram demonstrates a distribution around a mean.

31. **(B)** $(12x^2 + 6xy - 3xy^2) / (3xy) = \dfrac{12x^2}{3xy} + \dfrac{6xy}{3xy} - \dfrac{3xy^2}{3xy}$ Divide each term in the dividend by the divisor

$$= 4x + 2 - y$$

32. **(C)** Matt's age (x) is equal to 5 times Paul's age (p) minus 7.

33. **(D)** $t + 8 = 15$

$t + 8 - 8 = 15 - 8$

$t = 7$

34. **(C)** $|5x - 20| > 15$

$$x < \frac{-15 + 20}{5} \qquad x > \frac{15 + 20}{5}$$

$$x < \frac{5}{5} \qquad x > \frac{35}{5}$$

$$x < 1 \quad \text{or} \qquad x > 7$$

Since there is a lesser than connector, the connecting word is *or*, not *and*.

Science

1. **(C)** The number of protons is equal to the atomic number located on the periodic chart. Sodium (Na) has 11.

2. **(D)** The number of neutrons = atomic mass – atomic number.

3. **(C)** X-rays have the shortest wavelengths second only to gamma rays. Radio waves have long wavelengths and low frequencies.

4. **(C)** The person has a force of 50 N with a distance of 150 meters, so work done by the body is 50 × 150 = 7,500 joules.

5. **(B)** The active site is where an enzyme attaches to a substrate.

6. **(C)** Non-metals gain electrons easily and are poor conductors of electricity.

7. **(B)** The transitions metals have high conductivity, vivid colors, and a varied oxidation state.

8. **(D)** Strong bases will completely dissociate in solution and have stable cations. Weak bases partially dissociate. Water is considered neutral.

9. **(C)** Hydrocarbons have been discovered on planets within our solar system. The most common one is methane in lakes on Saturn's moon.

10. **(A)** In order for covalent bonding to occur there must be similar attractions of electrons between elements.

11. **(C)** Add 3KOH to the first molecule and then there will be 6H on the other side, so the second molecule will remain 1 and the equation is balanced for H_2O with 3 molecules of water.

12. **(A)** The density changes, not the volume displaced.

13. **(B)** Carbon dioxide converts directly from solid to gas dependent upon pressure, not temperature.

14. **(A)** This statement identifies the problem, suggests a direction to search for a solution, and makes a prediction.

15. **(A)** This statement is closest to a directional hypothesis.

16. **(B)** They know the problem and should start asking questions before reworking the hypothesis.

17. **(A)** This is a survey design. No intervention is being attempted; data is the only goal.

18. **(B)** dependent

19. **(D)** sleep, pain

20. **(C)** qualitative

21. **(B)** Deductive reasoning means working down from a theory.

22. **(C)** This is experimental.

23. **(D)** The best method will ensure that there is a randomized approach to control for extraneous variables or researcher bias.

24. **(A)** In the biological classification system, families are grouped under orders.

25. **(A)** A climate change might be the reason for an animal to develop blubber as an adaptation.

26. **(D)** In the provided grouping, RNA is a nucleic acid.

27. **(A)** The lysosomes remove cellular debris.

28. **(B)** Men have an X and Y chromosome.

29. **(B)** There will be four haploid cells resulting from meiosis.

30. **(B)** The cell membrane is replaced with a cell capsule in the bacterium.

31. **(B)** If a tall plant is crossed with a short plant, all the plants would be tall.

32. **(A)** Fever is the classical symptom of most infectious diseases.

33. **(B)** IgM is the antibody of a primary immune response.

34. **(C)** The father's genetic designation would be BB.

35. **(C)** Messenger RNA is the most important protein for DNA replication.

36. **(A)** The pericardium provides a barrier against infection.

37. **(C)** Medications that stimulate the sympathetic nervous system will cause an increased heart rate.

38. **(C)** The coronary venous blood drains directly into the right atrium.

39. **(A)** The sneeze is associated with irritation of the upper respiratory tract mucosa.

40. **(D)** The brain stem most likely controls respiration.

41. **(C)** The pulmonary stretch receptors decrease ventilatory rate and volume when stimulated.

42. **(A)** The keratinocytes are found in the epidermis of the skin.

43. **(A)** The loop of Henle is the only structure located in the nephron; the rest are outside of the structure.

44. **(C)** The renin-angiotensin system is activated when blood volume is low or there is a decrease in blood pressure.

45. **(B)** The kidneys activate intestinally absorbed Vitamin D.

46. **(B)** The corpus callosum connects the two cerebral hemispheres.

47. **(A)** Blockage of the cerebral aqueduct causes hydrocephalus.

48. **(C)** The spinothalamic tract is a sensory pathway of the spinal cord.

49. **(A)** The dura mater is the outermost membrane surrounding the brain.

50. **(B)** The brain receives about 20% of the cardiac output.

51. **(A)** The metabolic rate regulates insulin.

52. **(B)** Epinephrine is secreted by the adrenal medulla.

53. **(A)** Neutrophils are the type of white blood cell that account for the highest percentage.

54. **(A)** Eosinophils are the predominant phagocyte of early inflammation.

English and Language Usage

1. **(B)** This option alone identifies the word *longingly* included in the given sentence as an adjective. All other options are incorrect.

2. **(A)** This option correctly identifies *boys* as a subject and *harder* as an adverb.

3. **(B)** This option contains correct subject–verb agreement: "John and Joni… like." All other options contain incorrect subject–verb agreement with regard to number or case.

4. **(C)** This option contains correct subject–verb agreement: "eatery… offers" and "town… shows." All other options contain incorrect subject–verb agreement with regard to number.

5. **(B)** The antecedent, *Bob*, is singular and male, which means that *him* is the only correct answer. All other options are incorrect in either number, gender, or case.

6. **(C)** This option correctly completes the sentence. All other options are incorrect pronouns to use in this case.

7. **(A)** This option correctly contains double quotation marks around the whole quote. Option B contains quotations in the wrong places, option C has no quotation marks to properly indicate direct dialogue, and option D unnecessarily adds single quotes.

8. **(B)** This option correctly contains double quotation marks around the direct quote, and single quotes around the originally quoted question. Option A has no quotation marks to properly indicate direct dialogue, option C incorrectly places single quotes, and option D contains quotations in the wrong places.

9. **(C)** This option is an example of third-person point of view. Options A and B are examples of first-person point of view, and option D is an example of second-person point of view.

10. **(C)** This option is an example of first-person point of view. Option A is an example of second-person point of view. Options B and D are examples of third-person point of view.

11. **(C)** This option effectively uses transitional words to combine the sentences into a single sentence to reflect the original meaning of the group of sentences. All other options may lead to confusion of the writer's original intent.

12. **(D)** This option effectively uses transitional words to combine the sentences into a single sentence that still reflects the original meaning of the group of sentences.

13. **(B)** This option properly defines the word *coveting* (which has nothing to do with "cover," "concealing" or "cover up"). All other options are incorrect.

14. **(C)** This option correctly defines the word *macabre*. All other options are incorrect.

15. **(A)** The prefix *phyto-* originates from the Greek language. The word *phytonutrient* means "plant compound that benefits the body." Therefore, it can be concluded that this person was on the right path to good health.

16. **(C)** The suffix *-phobia* originates from the Greek language. The word *numerophobia* means "fear of numbers." Therefore, it can be concluded that this student was not enthusiastic about math or any subject where numbers are involved.

17. **(B)** This option is the correct spelling: *awesome* is a commonly misspelled word; its root word (*awe*) ends in a silent *e* which must be kept if the added suffix begins with a consonant as in *-some*.

18. **(B)** This option alone is spelled correctly. All other options are spelled incorrectly.

19. **(D)** This option contains the correct word to complete the given sentence. The clue "smoggy city" points to *emphysema* (a lung or respiratory problem).

20. **(B)** This option contains the only word set that completes the given sentence. *To, too,* and *two* are commonly misspelled and misused homophone (sound alike) words.

21. **(A)** This option is spelled correctly; *scarcely* is a commonly misspelled word. The adjective *barely* ("hardly, just, narrowly") offers a cue to identify *scarcely* as the correctly spelled word.

22. **(D)** This option is correct. All other options are commonly misspelled words: *affect* ("to alter something") is not *effect* ("the result of a cause"); *principal* ("chief" or "leader") is not *principle* ("belief" or "rule of conduct"); and *they're* (contraction of *they are*) is not *their* ("belonging to them").

23. **(A)** Because titles are not capitalized when following a name, the term *doctor* in this case is not capitalized and this is correct. All the other options contain capitalization errors.

24. **(D)** The word *Cotswolds* should be capitalized, as it is a geographical location and a proper noun in this context. There is no need to capitalize the words in options A, B, or C.

25. **(B)** This option is correctly punctuated with a semicolon separating two independent clauses.

26. **(C)** To punctuate this sentence, parentheses would be correct because the supplementary or explanatory material occurs within a sentence.

27. **(B)** This option is constructed as a simple sentence containing one subject and a compound verb. Although the sentence has modifiers, there are no clauses adding to the complexity of the sentence structure, as is the case in the other options.

28. **(D)** This option is constructed as a simple sentence with one subject and a compound verb. Although the sentence is detailed, there are no clauses adding to the complexity of the sentence structure, as in the case of all other options.

29. **(C)** This option makes one clause subordinate to the other by the addition of a subordinating conjunction. Options A and B contain two clauses of equal weight, and option C has the opposite focus.

30. **(A)** This option completes the sentence as a simple sentence. All other options are examples of compound sentences.

31. **(D)** This option clearly and succinctly conveys the writer's intent to accurately describe the woman. The writing in the other options could lead to confusion.

32. **(D)** This option is an example of grammar used to enhance clarity and readability. The four sentences are combined into one clear, succinct sentence that is easy to read and understand. The other options, while employing correct grammar to condense the four sentences, do not do so in a manner that clearly expresses the writer's intent.

33. **(C)** This option effectively uses transitional words to combine the sentences into a single sentence that still reflects the original meaning of the group of sentences.

34. **(C)** This option effectively uses transitional words to combine the sentences into a single sentence that still reflects the original meaning of the group of sentences.

NOTES

NOTES

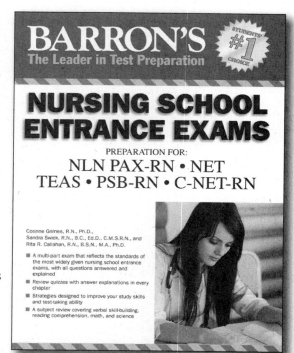
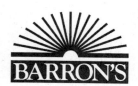

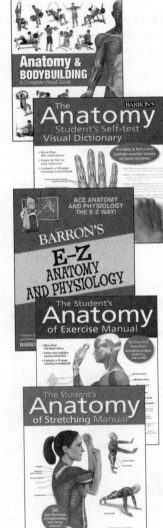

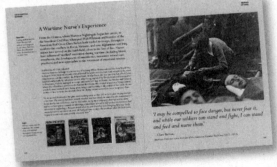
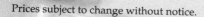

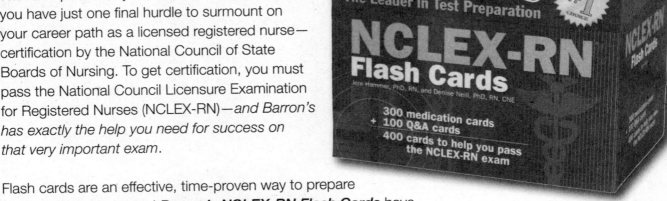
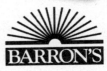
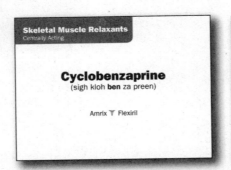
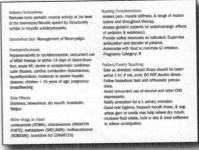